# Wheat-Free, Gluten-Free
# Cookbook for Kids
# and Busy Adults

•

## Second Edition

•

## Connie Sarros

New York  Chicago  San Francisco  Lisbon  London  Madrid  Mexico City
Milan  New Delhi  San Juan  Seoul  Singapore  Sydney  Toronto

The *McGraw·Hill* Companies

**Library of Congress Cataloging-in-Publication Data**

Sarros, Connie.
    Wheat-free, gluten-free cookbook for kids and busy adults / by Connie Sarros. —
2nd ed.
        p.    cm.
    Includes index.
    ISBN-13: 978-0-07-162747-4 (alk. paper)
    ISBN-10: 0-07-162747-2 (alk. paper)
    1. Wheat-free diet—Recipes.    2. Gluten-free diet—Recipes.    3. Children—
Nutrition.    4. Quick and easy cookery.    I. Title.

    RM237.87.S268    2009
    641.5'63—dc22                                                            2009004715

2  3  4  5  6  7  8  9  10  11  12  13  14  15  16  17  18  19  20  21  22  23  24    DOC/DOC    0

ISBN    978-0-07-162747-4
MHID      0-07-162747-2

Interior design by Sue Hartman
Interior illustrations by Jacqueline Dubé and Dean Stanton, Birch Design Studios

McGraw-Hill books are available at special quantity discounts to use as premiums and sales promotions or for use in corporate training programs. To contact a representative please e-mail us at bulksales@mcgraw-hill.com.

*I dedicate this book to four very important groups of people.*

*First, this book is dedicated to all the young children with celiac disease or autism. You deserve to have fun in the kitchen making foods that are easy to prepare and fun to eat.*

*Second, this book is dedicated to busy adults who want to prepare and provide nourishing meals but don't have a lot of time to spend in the kitchen.*

*Third, a special "thank-you" to my editor, Fiona Sarne, and all of the people at McGraw-Hill who helped publish this book. I thank you not only for your help and guidance, but for recognizing the need for special-diet cookbooks.*

*Finally, I dedicate this book to my family, who urged me to pursue this venture. Their love and support helped to make this book a reality.*

# Contents

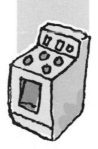

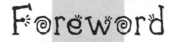

# Foreword

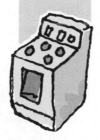

Celiac disease is a syndrome characterized by damage of the small intestinal mucosa caused by the gliadin found in wheat gluten and other similar alcohol-soluble proteins, such as barley and rye, in genetically susceptible persons. The consumption of gluten in these persons leads to a self-perpetuating mucosal damage, while the elimination of gluten from the diet results in a full mucosal recovery. The clinical manifestations of celiac disease are protean in nature and vary markedly with the age of the patient, the duration and extent of disease, and the presence of symptoms occurring outside of the intestines. In addition to the classic gastrointestinal form, a variety of other clinical manifestations of celiac disease have been described, including atypical and asymptomatic forms. While in the past, celiac disease was typically considered a pediatric condition, we now are aware that the disease may become clinically evident after years of silent intestinal damage following exposure to gluten. Therefore, the diagnosis of celiac disease can be extremely challenging and currently relies on a sensitive and specific algorithm that allows the identification of different manifestations of the disease. Blood tests developed in the last decade provide a noninvasive tool to screen both individuals at risk for the disease and the general population. However, the current gold standard for the diagnosis of celiac disease remains the upper endoscopy.

The keystone treatment of celiac disease patients is a lifelong elimination diet in which food products containing gluten are avoided. While in principle the treatment appears simple and straightforward, embracing a gluten-free diet is not an easy enterprise. There are things in life that we do automatically without paying attention to them: How many times have we driven back home from work thinking about something else and found ourselves at the garage door without recalling how we got there? How often have we performed routine tasks such as tied our shoes, brushed our teeth, and listened to sounds of nature and yet didn't have distinct memory of these acts later? For the vast majority of human beings, eating is another automatic activity, but not so for celiacs, for whom eating is a very energy-consuming task of their daily routine. A fair amount of mental, physical, and social energy is devoted to what should be one of life's most natural and enjoyable activities. In the United States, this task has been aggravated in the past by the limited alternatives to food containing gluten. All this translates into a monumental undertaking, particularly for those who have to please the taste of celiac children. To make the endeavor even more challenging, the fast-lane lifestyle typical of our society, including our fast-food habit, cannot be applied to the celiac cuisine. With this book, Ms. Sarros gives us the tools to address these challenges, with a creative approach that brings the task of preparing food for celiac kids and working adults back to human dimensions. The book is fresh, easy to follow, and most important, full of "humorous condiment." Reading through her recipes, you discover such a bottom-line simplicity to cooking gluten-free that you find yourself asking, "That's it?"

—Alessio Fasano, M.D.
University of Maryland Center for Celiac Research

# Preface

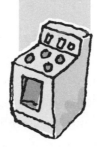

## Eating Gluten-Free

Eating gluten-free means that you can still enjoy all of your favorite foods just by changing a few of the ingredients. If you're on a gluten-free diet, you should never eat anything that contains or comes in direct contact with wheat, rye, or barley. Pure oats are gluten-free, which means that they are grown in dedicated fields, where no wheat, rye, or barley are grown, and are processed in dedicated facilities, where there are no glutinous grains processed. Many celiacs can tolerate pure oats, but some cannot. If you see any of the following terms in a list of ingredients, it means that the food is *not* gluten-free:

Abyssinian hard wheat (*Triticum durum*)
All-purpose flour
Barley (or *Hordeum*)
Beer
Bouillon (some)
Bran
Broth (some)

Bulgur

Coffee creamer substitute (most are gluten-free)

Couscous

Cracker meal

Durum

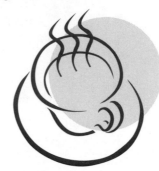

Einkorn wheat

Farina

Flavored instant coffee (some)

Flavored instant tea (some)

Fu (dried wheat gluten)

Gelatinized starch (read the label ingredients; this frequently contains wheat, but not always)

Gluten

Graham flour

Granary flour

Gravy mixes (most gravy mixes are made with wheat)

Groat

Hamburger patties (both commercially packaged frozen hamburger patties and those served in restaurants and fast-food outlets may contain wheat-based fillers; read the ingredients on the package or ask whether prepared hamburger is gluten-free)

Hydrolyzed plant protein (HPP)

Hydrolyzed vegetable protein (HVP)

Job's tears (aka pearl barley)

Kamut (or kawmut)

Malt

Malt vinegar

Natural flavoring (this may or may not contain wheat or barley; read the ingredients on the label)

Rice malt (contains barley or koji, which is used to make sake)

Rice syrup (check the label: most is gluten-free, but a few brands may contain barley malt enzymes)

Rye

Sausage (some contain wheat fillers)

Seitan

Semolina

Shoyu

Soba noodles

Soy sauce (many)

Spelt (or *spelta*)

Starch (starch processed in the United States and Canada is
    usually made from cornstarch; this is not the case in
    many other countries)

Suet in packets

Teriyaki sauce (many)

Triticale

*Triticum*

Udon (wheat noodles)

Vitamins (some contain gluten)

White flour

Wholemeal flour

## Eating Dairy-Free

In putting together this revised edition, I thought it was important to highlight dairy-free, or casein-free, alternatives. Research-
ers, physicians, and parents are beginning to discover, in a growing
number of cases, that a dairy-free, gluten-free diet can help man-
age many conditions. Although gluten-free diets are primarily
intended for those who have celiac disease, combining them with
dairy-free alternatives may help conditions like autism signifi-
cantly. Dr. Jerry Kartzinel, who works with autistic children,
believes that eating wheat and dairy acts as an opiate in the brains
of children with autism, altering their behavior, perceptions, and
responses to their environment. Jenny McCarthy's book *Louder*

## Who Benefits from a Gluten-Free, Dairy-Free Diet?

A gluten- and dairy-free diet is believed to help people not only with food allergies, celiac disease, and autism but also those with the following conditions:

ADHD (attention deficit/hyperactivity disorder)

Aggression

ALS (amyotrophic lateral sclerosis; often referred to as Lou Gehrig's disease)

Anxiety

Bulimia nervosa

Chronic fatigue syndrome/fibromyalgia

Dementia in those under seventy years old

Depression

Dermatitis

Developmental delays

Diabetes mellitus (Types I and II)

Diverticulitis

Down syndrome

Epilepsy

Gait disturbances

Headaches

IBS (irritable bowel syndrome)

Infertility

Inflammatory bowel syndrome

Intestinal lymphoma

Maldigestion/malabsorption

Osteoporosis

Panic attacks

PDD (pervasive developmental disorder)

Pernicious anemia

Psoriasis

Rheumatoid arthritis

Schizophrenia
Sjogren's syndrome
Stomach ulcers
Systemic lupus
Thyroid problems

Before you consider a change in your or your child's diet, though, consult with a physician and dietitian to ensure adequate nutrition.

*Than Words: A Mother's Journey in Healing Autism* describes the dramatic improvement in her son's behavior on the gluten free, dairy-free diet. There is significant evidence that the diet is helpful in lessening autistic symptoms, such as impulsive behaviors, lack of focus, and even speech problems.

Before you consider a change in your or your child's diet, consult with a physician and dietitian to make sure your diet provides adequate nutrition.

When you are dairy-free, you need to be aware of all the different words on labels that mean that dairy is included. Milk-based products have two main components: *lactose* is the sugar in milk; *casein* is the protein in milk. Casein helps to bind foods together, so it is often hidden in food—even in packages labeled "dairy free."

If you see any of the following listed on a package, it means the product contains lactose or casein and, therefore, is not dairy-free:

Acidophilus milk
Amylase
Artificial butter flavor
*Avena* (this is often processed with milk)
Bouillon cubes or powder (some)

Broths (some are processed with milk)

Butter

Buttermilk

Calcium caseinate

Caramel coloring
     (may contain lactose)

Casein

Caseinates

Cheese

Chorizo (commercial brands
     may contain casein; "milk"
     will be listed in the ingredients)

Cottage cheese

Cream

Curds

Delactosed whey

Dextrin (used as a thickening agent in some pharmaceuticals
     and candy, it is dairy- and gluten-free if made in the
     United States and Canada)

Galactose

Ghee

Ginger ale

Glutamic acid

Goats' milk

Horseradish

Hot dogs (many contain casein and/or wheat)

Lactalbumin

Lactalbumin phosphate

Lactic acid (may or may not contain milk)

Lactoglobulin

Lactose

Lactulose

Lunch meats (some contain casein)

Magnesium caseinate

Margarine (some are dairy-free)

Milk

Miso (soybean paste fermented with barley, rice, or other grain)

Monosodium glutamate or MSG (brands made outside the United States)

Nondairy creamer and butter

Nondairy whipped toppings (most)

Pepperoni

Pickles (some)

Potassium caseinate

Rennet casein

Root beer

Salami

Sauerkraut (some)

Sausage (many contain casein)

Soy cheeses (many)

Sulfites

Vegetable broths or bouillon (most)

Whey

Yogurt

The following ingredients may contain milk protein:

Bavarian cream flavoring

Brown sugar flavoring

Coconut cream flavoring

Natural chocolate flavoring

Natural flavorings sometimes have hidden ingredients that contain gluten and/or casein. The FDA (Food and Drug Administration) has passed rules in recent years that make the labeling on foods easier to understand. If a product contains any dairy or wheat, it now has to be clearly stated in the list of ingredients, making it so much easier to identify which foods are safe to eat for celiacs and those with autism.

## Labels on Food Packages

Because of kosher dietary laws, many food packages are marked with letters that make it easier to recognize foods that contain dairy:

"D" on a label, next to "K" or "U" means that milk protein (casein) is present.

"P" on a label stands for "parve," meaning it is dairy-free.

## Milk

Fortunately, there are many types of nondairy milk that taste good and are excellent to use when cooking. Here are some great examples:

Almond milk
Coconut milk
Hemp milk
Rice milk
Soy milk (some brands contain casein)
Vanilla rice milk
Vanilla soy milk (some brands contain casein)

If you need to use powdered or dry milk, a good product to use is DariFree milk powder (made from potatoes), which is both dairy- and gluten-free.

For recipes that call for sweetened condensed milk, you can make your own:

## Dairy-Free Sweetened Condensed Milk

4 ounces dairy-free silken tofu
¼ cup dairy-free vanilla soy milk
¼ cup sugar or maple syrup

1. Put the tofu, soy milk, and sugar or maple syrup in a blender.
2. Blend until smooth.

**Note:** Depending on your taste, you may want to add additional sugar or maple syrup. For a thinner consistency, add more soy milk. For a thicker consistency, add more tofu.

## Margarines and Spreads

In recent years, margarines and spreads that are gluten-free and dairy-free have become more readily available. There should be a "P" on the labels or packaging to indicate that the product is parve (dairy-free). Here is a list of some gluten-free and dairy-free margarines and spreads:

Earth Balance
Fleischmann's Light Margarine
Hain Safflower Oil Margarine
Mother's Margarine
Nucoa Margarine
Parkay margarine
Shedd's Willow Run Soybean Margarine
Smart Balance
Spectrum Spread (by Spectrum Foods)

## A Smart Dairy-Free Diet

Dairy products contain some pretty important things that your body needs, like calcium, protein, phosphorous, and vitamin D. It's important to eat other foods that also have these nutrients.

You can get your calcium from dark, leafy green vegetables, like spinach, kale, and collard greens. You can also get calcium from seafood, especially shellfish and salmon. The amount of calcium that is actually absorbed into the body from these foods may not be ample, so it may be advisable to take calcium supplements. For protein, you can get most of what you need from beans, like white beans, navy beans, and chickpeas. Casein-free tofu is also packed with protein. For stronger teeth and bones, you need to find a way to replace the phosphorous that's found in milk. Fortunately, you can find phosphorous in foods like meat, fish, and beans. Are you getting enough vitamin D? Did you know that sunlight stimulates the body to produce vitamin D? Just ten to fifteen minutes in direct sunlight each day will give your body the amount of vitamin D it needs. This vitamin can also be found in many cereals, fish, and oysters.

Young cooks who are not sure if certain ingredients are safe for their diet should ask an adult before using them.

Brand names are listed throughout this book to help you find gluten-free and/or dairy-free products. Companies change their recipes, methods of production, and suppliers, so it is still necessary to read labels each time you purchase a product. The brand names listed are, at the time of the printing of this book, gluten- and/or dairy-free in the United States. However, these same brands may not be gluten- and/or dairy-free in Canada or other countries. For example, Lea and Perrins Worcestershire Sauce distributed in the United States is gluten-free. Lea and Perrins Worcestershire Sauce sold in Canada has malt added and is, therefore, not gluten-free. Always read labels.

# Cooking Basics

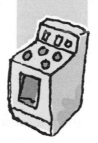

**i**'ve made sure that the recipes in this book are easy to prepare! There are no fancy gadgets required, and none of the recipes require the use of a mixer, though a few do use a blender. (Remember to put the lid on the blender before turning it on!)

Adult supervision will be needed with some of the recipes, especially when sharp knives are used to chop ingredients or hot pans need to come out of the oven.

Because children differ in age and ability and adults may only have limited time available for culinary creations, the recipes in this book offer simple-to-prepare foods that all age groups will enjoy!

## Notes About Kitchen Ingredients

It is assumed that only gluten-free brands of products will be purchased. Dairy-free alternatives are listed along with suggested dairy-free brand names for each recipe calling for dairy. All products need not be both gluten- and dairy-free for those who are not on a dairy-free diet. Remember to read labels each time you buy something to be sure it is still gluten- and/or dairy-free.

- **Cocoa.** When cocoa is listed as an ingredient of a recipe, you should use dry, unsweetened cocoa powder, not a hot chocolate mix.
- **Dark chocolate.** Only dark chocolate is used in this cookbook, since milk chocolate contains dairy. Many brands of semisweet chocolate chips are also dairy-free. Be sure to read labels to make sure the dark chocolate or semisweet chocolate you purchase is dairy-free if you cannot tolerate dairy.
- **Melting chocolate in the microwave.** A few of the recipes direct you to melt chocolate in the microwave. The easiest way to do this is to break the chocolate into smaller pieces, then place the pieces in a glass bowl. Place the bowl in the microwave and heat on high for 1 minute. Take the bowl out, stir the chocolate, then place the bowl back into the microwave and continue to cook, taking it out every 30 seconds to stir the mixture. As soon as most of the chocolate is melted, remove it from the microwave and stir the mix until all of the chocolate has melted completely. Overcooking the chocolate will cause it to turn into a hardened mush that can't easily be used in recipes, so watch it closely. Use a pot holder when removing the bowl from the microwave because the bowl may get quite hot.
- **Natural ingredients.** The ingredients in this book are mostly natural. There are a few exceptions. Dairy-free margarine is listed in a few recipes where oil or some other natural butter substitute cannot be used successfully. Even margarine can be all-natural when you use organic shortening or Earth Balance (a natural, nondairy spread). Occasionally, a premixed package of dry soup or seasoning is used for ease of preparation.
- **Nonstick spray.** Many of the commercial nonstick cooking sprays are gluten- and dairy-free. Be aware that some contain

wheat flour; this will be clearly marked on the label and in the list of ingredients.

    ● **Soy cheese.** Cheese made from soy is often used as a dairy-free substitute for dairy cheese. Many of the soy products, however, contain casein. Fortunately, there are some excellent varieties of vegan cheeses available; many taste good and melt well.

    ● **Soy milk and rice milk.** Some varieties of soy and rice milk are lactose-free; some are lactose- and casein-free. Read the labels carefully.

# Meal Planning

Planning a meal is like painting a picture. Think about having different colors and textures on the plate, and of course think about nutrition.

    Some people (both kids and adults) crinkle their noses when they hear the word "vegetables" . . . but vegetables can be delicious . . . really! Both lunch and dinner should include vegetables. Think of all of the fun ways to add veggies to a meal—in a salad, as a cooked side dish, as part of a stew, or in a casserole. For lunches, veggies can be added to soups, cut into strips and served with a dip, or added to a sandwich or wrap. Preparing cooked vegetables can be as easy as steaming them in a little bit of water. This list includes vegetables that are delicious steamed:

Asparagus
Broccoli
Brussels sprouts
Butter beans
Cabbage
Carrots

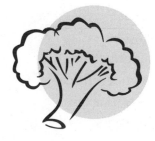

Corn
Green beans
Italian green beans
Lima beans
Peas
Snow peas
Spinach
Sweet potatoes or yams
White potatoes
Zucchini

Another way to get creative is to make a salad using different kinds of lettuce and greens. Keep in mind that the darker the green, the better it is for you. Here is just a sampling of different varieties of greens you can use:

Arugula
Bibb lettuce
Butterhead lettuce
Cabbage
Dandelion greens (not the ones from your yard that have
    been sprayed with chemicals, but the natural or organic
    kind found at the grocery store)
Endive
Iceberg lettuce
Leaf lettuce
Mesclun greens
Mustard greens
Radicchio
Red leaf lettuce
Romaine lettuce
Spinach leaves
Watercress

Along with greens, it's fun to add all kinds of other things to salads:

Artichoke hearts
Beets
Bell peppers
Black beans
Broccoli
Carrots
Cauliflower
Celery
Cheese (vegan cheese if you are dairy-free)
Corn
Cucumbers
Garbanzo beans
Gluten-free croutons
Green beans
Green onions
Hearts of palm
Kidney beans
Mushroom slices
Olives
Onion slices
Peas
Peperoncini
Radishes
Sunflower seeds
Tomatoes
Walnuts
Zucchini

When planning a meal, think about how much time you have to prepare it. Some of the meals in this book take 30 minutes or less to prepare. Others can be put together ahead of time, covered and kept in the refrigerator, then baked just before dinner (for the days when you'll be getting home late). Some of the recipes use five ingredients or less (for those times when the pantry is bare). And some are easy enough that the very young can make them unassisted.

## Kitchen Hints

The following hints will help you to be organized and safe in the kitchen:

- Children should ask an adult for permission before cooking any recipe.
- Children should ask an adult to help when a recipe calls for using a microwave, stove, oven, sharp knife, scissors, grater, peeler, or any electrical appliance.
- Read through the entire recipe before you begin cooking to make sure you understand the directions and that you have all the ingredients and utensils that will be needed.
- Measure all the ingredients before you begin mixing them.
- Wash fresh fruits, vegetables, meats, and fish in cold water before preparing the recipe.
- Wash your hands with antibacterial soap before you begin cooking, when you are finished cooking, and immediately after handling fresh meat, poultry, or fish.
- Before you start mixing the ingredients, be sure you have enough time to make the recipe. Some recipes cook in an electric slow cooker for as long as 8 hours, which means you will need to assemble your dinner in the morning. Others need to be refrigerated for several hours before serving or marinated for a few hours before cooking.

- Use metal or aluminum pans when baking cookies and breads. The dark-coated pans will cause your baked goods to burn on the bottom.
- Use only pans that are the size called for in the recipe. Using the right size pan ensures that your foods will bake evenly.
- Be very careful when opening cans. The cut edges on the can and on the lid are very sharp.
- When cooking on the stove, turn all pot handles away from you so the pots won't be knocked over accidentally.
- If you are making a sticky batter, spread or pat the batter into the baking pan evenly with a wet spatula or dampened hands.
- Use thick, dry pot holders to handle all hot pots, pans, casseroles, and baking sheets.
- Clean the countertops and utensils as you use them.
- Wipe floor spills as soon as they happen. Keeping floors clean prevents you and others in the kitchen from slipping.
- Don't lift the lid from a slow cooker while cooking, especially during the first three quarters of the cooking time. The heat lost during a quick peek could add 30 minutes to the cooking time.
- In an electric slow cooker, vegetables take longer to cook than meat, so place the vegetables on the bottom of the pot.
- After you serve your food, your pan may be crusted and difficult to clean. Put a few drops of dish soap in the pan, and add warm water. Then let the pan soak awhile. The stuck-on food should clean off easily after soaking.

## Cooking Techniques
**Baking:** When baking, place food on the center rack in the oven, unless otherwise stated in the recipe. Leave at least 2 inches of space around the pan. Overcrowding in the oven causes uneven cooking. Most baked items will cook in the amount of time

indicated in each recipe. However, ovens vary, so check the baked item about 5 minutes before it should be done to see if it is cooked through so it doesn't dry out or burn. There are times you will have to leave something baking longer than indicated in the recipe. To test whether cakes, muffins, and sweet breads are done baking, insert a toothpick in the center and pull it back out. If it comes out dry, the product is done cooking.

**Boiling Over:** Before you steam rice or boil pasta, butter the rim of the pot. This will help keep the water from boiling over.

**Cakes:** To keep a cake fresh longer, place half an apple in the cake container when you store it.

**Candy:** Try to make your candy on dry days. Candy does not set as well on humid or rainy days.

**Casseroles:** Most casseroles may be assembled up to 24 hours in advance and refrigerated. Some casserole containers, like those made of Pyrex and stainless steel, can be placed in a hot, pre-heated oven right out of the refrigerator. Other cold containers, like glass dishes, must be placed in a cold oven before the heat is turned on. (When a cold glass dish is placed in a cold oven, the dish will warm slowly as the oven heats, preventing the glass from shattering.)

**Cheese:** There are two basic kinds of vegan cheeses—one that melts easily and one that does not. In cold dishes, it doesn't make any difference which of these cheeses you use, but in recipes that are cooked, the melting kind of cheese is preferable. The package will clearly state, "It melts!"

**Chopping, Cutting, Grating:** Preparing ingredients often requires chopping, cutting, or grating one or more ingredients. Depending on the age of the chef, it may be necessary for an adult to help with these sorts of tasks. If children are grating, remind them that the grater has sharp holes and they should guard against scraping their fingertips or knuckles against the holes.

**Cookies:** To keep cookies soft, place a slice of soft, gluten-free bread in the storage container with them. To prevent cookies from spreading while baking, refrigerate the dough on the baking sheet for 30 minutes before baking. If you want your cookies to have the same size and appearance, use a small ice-cream scoop or a melon baller to spoon out the cookie dough (depending on how large or small you want to make the cookies). This method also keeps your fingers clean. Dip the scoop in warm water frequently to keep the dough from sticking to it. Some cookies may not brown much, so you can't always judge when a cookie is baked through by the color on the outside. Touch the top of the cookie lightly with your finger; if no imprint remains, then the cookie is baked through.

**Dash:** Whenever a measurement is less than ⅛ teaspoon, the recipe will call for a "dash." To add a dash, sprinkle in just a tiny amount of the ingredient.

**"Diet," "Low Calorie," and "Lite" Ingredients:** Some of the recipes in this book list mayonnaise and cola or soda in the ingredients. Do not use the light or diet versions of these products. Often the diet versions will break down when heated (in an oven or microwave, or on top of the stove in a pan) and will leave a dreadful metallic taste.

**Eggs:** The shell of a fresh egg is rough and chalky looking. An old egg will have a shell that is smooth and shiny. Another way to check an egg's freshness is to place the egg in a pot of cold, salted water. If the egg sinks, it is fresh. If it floats, it is not fresh, so throw it away! If you see any red specks in an egg, throw it out. When a recipe calls for eggs to be separated (meaning egg whites and egg yolks will be used separately), this is easier to do when the eggs are cold.

**Flour Mixture:** Recipes in most cookbooks direct you to "sift the flour." The recipes in this cookbook are designed to be easy, so no sifting of flour is needed. When measuring the various flours to make the initial batch of gluten-free flour mixture, you will need to sift or whisk the ingredients to blend them thoroughly; but sifting small amounts of the mixture for use in individual recipes is not necessary. When measuring the amount of the gluten-free flour mixture needed in a recipe, do not pack the flour into the measuring cup. Lightly spoon the flour mixture into the cup, then level it off with the side of a knife. Frequently you will be directed to mix all the dry ingredients together with a wire whisk; this is to incorporate a little air into the mixture in place of sifting.

**Frozen Vegetables:** A quick way to separate frozen vegetables to use in a casserole is to put the vegetables in a colander, then set the colander in the sink under hot running water. Another method is to place the frozen vegetables in a glass bowl and microwave them on high for 2 to 3 minutes (the length of time depends on the kind of vegetable and the quantity being thawed).

**Fudge:** Always use a wooden spoon when making fudge. (A metal spoon may cause the mixture to taste grainy.)

**Gelatin Molds:** To remove gelatin salads or desserts from molds more easily, lightly brush the mold with oil or spray it with nonstick spray before pouring in the mixture.

**Juicing Citrus Fruits:** To get the most juice out of fresh lemons, limes, and oranges, bring them to room temperature, then roll them under your palm against the kitchen countertop before squeezing. If you don't have time to let the fruit come to room temperature, cut it in half, set it on a plate, and microwave it for a few seconds.

**Margarine:** Dairy-free margarine is available in sticks (like butter) and in tubs. For many dessert recipes, it is important to use the stick margarine because the mixture that comes in tubs contains too much water. The high water content in the tubs can negatively affect the outcome of your dessert.

**Marshmallows:** Even though most commercial brands of marshmallows are both gluten- and dairy-free, specific brand names are included in ingredients lists throughout this book.

**Measurements:** Dry products should be measured using a nested measuring cup—instead of a large measuring cup with multiple measuring lines—so the top can be leveled off with a knife. When measuring brown sugar, pack it down into the cup as tightly as possible. Never pack down any flour or powdered sugar; instead, lightly spoon it into the measuring cup. Liquids should be measured in a glass measuring cup. To get the correct reading, set the glass cup on the counter and stoop down so the measuring line is at eye level.

**Measuring Corn Syrup, Molasses, and Honey:** Before you measure sticky ingredients like corn syrup, molasses, or honey, dip the measuring cup or spoon in hot water or spray it with gluten-free nonstick cooking spray, which will help prevent sticking and make it easier to pour out the measured ingredient.

**Nutritional Facts:** Nutritional information is listed for each recipe in this book, calculated from the National Data Laboratory of the Agricultural Research Service, nal.usda.gov/fnic/foodcomp/search. When appropriate, recipes offer suggestions for dairy-free ingredients, however, these ingredients are *not* reflected in nutritional breakdowns. Recipes using milk give nutritional counts based on whole milk; 1 percent milk may be used in place of whole milk to reduce the amount of fat in a recipe. There are two recipes in this book for gluten-free flour mixtures; nutritional counts throughout this book are based on the Basic Gluten-Free Flour Mixture ingredients.

**Pancakes:** Use a turkey baster to squeeze your pancake batter onto the hot griddle. You'll get perfectly shaped pancakes every time.

**Potatoes:** Most of the recipes in this book do not direct you to peel the potatoes. Much of the nutritional value of a potato is found in its skin. Be sure to wash the outside of the potato before cooking.

**Preheating the Oven:** Turn on the oven about 10 minutes before you bake anything so it can reach the preset temperature. The exception, as stated earlier, is when you are baking a casserole or other food that was prepared in a glass dish and has been refrigerated; in this case, start with a cold oven.

**Temperature for Baking:** Do not increase the oven temperature above that recommended in the recipe. It won't speed up the cooking process. Your product will burn on the outside, and it won't be cooked on the inside.

**Wooden Skewers:** When using wooden skewers for kabobs, soak them in cold water for 30 minutes before stringing foods. Soaking prevents skewers from burning during cooking.

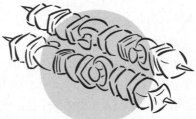

## Measurements

1 tablespoon = 3 teaspoons

1 fluid ounce = 2 tablespoons

1 jigger = 3 tablespoons

¼ cup = 4 tablespoons

⅓ cup = 5⅓ tablespoons

½ cup = 8 tablespoons

1 cup = ½ pint = 16 tablespoons

1 cup = 8 fluid ounces

1 pint = 2 cups

1 quart = 4 cups = 2 pints

½ gallon = 2 quarts

1 gallon = 4 quarts

½ stick butter = 4 tablespoons = ¼ cup

1 stick butter = 8 tablespoons = ½ cup

1 pound butter = 4 sticks = 2 cups

1 pound = 16 ounces

1 pound granulated sugar = 2¼ cups

1 pound brown sugar = 2¼ cups, packed down

1 pound confectioners' sugar = 3½ cups, sifted

1 square baking chocolate = 1 ounce

# Gluten-Free Flour Mixtures

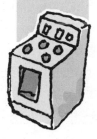

aking can be so much fun when you experiment with different flour mixtures. There is no single alternative flour that can duplicate the taste and texture of wheat flour, but fortunately, when different gluten-free flours are blended together, they can imitate wheat flour almost exactly.

Each type of gluten-free flour has its own properties that add something to the flour mixture. Here is a list of some of the gluten-free flours available:

Acorn flour
Almond flour
Amaranth flour
Brown rice flour
Buckwheat flour
Chestnut flour
Coconut flour
Corn flour
Fava bean flour
Garbanzo bean flour (or chickpea flour)

Lentil flour

Mesquite flour

Millet flour

Montina flour (a commercially available gluten-free flour
   blend)

Mung bean flour

Oat flour (made from pure, uncontaminated oats)

Pea flour

Potato flour (used like cornstarch to thicken)

Potato starch (used in flour mixtures for baking)

Quinoa flour

Sorghum flour

Soy flour

Sweet potato flour

Sweet rice flour (used like cornstarch to thicken)

Tapioca flour

Teff flour

White rice flour

If you combine flours in different amounts, you will get varied results. That's why it's important, when making recipes from a gluten-free and/or dairy-free cookbook, that you use the flour mixture recommended. If you use a different flour mixture from what is recommended, it may alter the outcome of your pastry or bread.

Following are two gluten-free flour mixtures. One is standard and basic; the other has more fiber. Both recipes will work equally well with the recipes in this book. If you choose to make more than one recipe of the flour mixture at a time, measure and sift the first batch into a large bowl, then measure and sift the second batch into the same bowl. Use a wire whisk to blend the two batches thoroughly. Spoon the flour mixture into a large, self-seal freezer bag and store it in the freezer to keep it fresh. When you are ready to bake, measure out the amount you need, then let it stand for 15 minutes to come to room temperature.

Both flour mixtures call for xanthan gum. This ingredient is not included in most commercial gluten-free baking mixes, so most recipes in other gluten-free cookbooks list the gum as one of the ingredients to be added when you bake. Xanthan gum is a white powder that is sold in a pouch or a jar. Adding a small amount of this gum will help keep your baked goods from crumbling. If you make a recipe from another cookbook that calls for the gum to be added and you are using one of the flour mixtures in this book, it is not necessary to add the additional gum listed in the recipe. While it is highly recommended that you use one of the following flour mixtures when making the recipes in this cookbook, if you choose to use a different flour mixture, you will need to add xanthan gum to your mixture:

- **Cookies**: add ⅛ to ¼ teaspoon xanthan gum per 1 cup of flour
- **Cake:** add ¼ to ½ teaspoon xanthan gum per 1 cup of flour
- **Bread:** add ¾ to 1 teaspoon xanthan gum per 1 cup of flour

Many recipes in this book list "gluten-free flour mixture" in the ingredients. The nutritional facts that follow each recipe are based on baking with the Basic Gluten-Free Flour Mixture, but as already stated, you may also use the High-Fiber, Gluten-Free Flour Mixture, which will provide additional fiber.

## ꓭasic Gluten-Free Flour Mixture

2½ cups rice flour

1 cup potato starch

1 cup sorghum flour

1 cup tapioca flour

¼ cup cornstarch

¼ cup garbanzo bean flour

2 tablespoons xanthan gum

Sift all the ingredients into a bowl, then whisk them with a wire whisk to assure that everything is blended evenly.

*Makes 6 cups*

Per ¼ cup—Calories: 119; Total fat: 0.3 g; Saturated fat: 0 g; Cholesterol: 0 mg; Sodium: 1 mg; Carbohydrates: 27.2 g; Fiber: 1.4 g; Sugar: 0.1 g; Protein: 1.1 g

## ꓧigh-Fiber, Gluten-Free Flour Mixture

This mixture has 4.12 grams of fiber per ¼ cup flour mixture.

2½ cups brown rice flour

1½ cups sorghum flour

1 cup potato starch

1 cup tapioca flour

1 cup coconut flour

¾ cup garbanzo bean flour

⅔ cup golden flaxseed meal

¼ cup cornstarch

3 tablespoons xanthan gum

Sift all the ingredients into a bowl, then whisk them with a wire whisk to assure that everything is blended evenly.

*Makes 7¾ cups*

Per ¼ cup—Calories: 142; Total fat: 1.6 g; Saturated fat: 0.2 g; Cholesterol: 0 mg; Sodium: 1 mg; Carbohydrates: 29.1 g; Fiber: 4.12 g; Sugar: 0.08 g; Protein: 2.9 g

# 1

# Snacks

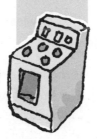

## Spicy Cheesy Spread

1 cup grated cheddar cheese (Vegan Gourmet Cheddar Cheese
   Alternative is dairy-free)
2 tablespoons canned, chopped green chilies
¼ cup mayonnaise
¼ teaspoon chili powder
2½ ounces (about 60) gluten-free tortilla chips (Frito Lay Tostitos
   Bite Size Rounds Tortilla Chips are gluten-free)

1. Preheat broiler.
2. In a bowl, stir together the grated cheese with the chilies, mayonnaise, and chili powder. Use a knife to spread the cheese mixture over the tortilla chips.
3. Place the chips on a baking sheet. Broil about 3 minutes or just until the cheese is slightly toasted.

*Makes 20 (3-chip) servings*

One serving—Calories: 41; Total fat: 2.4 g; Saturated fat: 0.3 g; Cholesterol: 0.7 mg;
Sodium: 72 mg; Carbohydrates: 4.4 g; Fiber: 0.1 g; Sugar: 0.2 g; Protein: 0.7 g

# Taco Dip

1½ tablespoons olive oil

2 green onions, sliced thin

1 (16-ounce) can refried beans

¼ cup water

¼ cup salsa

¾ cup shredded cheddar cheese (Vegan Gourmet Cheddar Cheese
   Alternative is dairy-free)

1. In a small saucepan, heat the oil for 10 seconds.
2. Add the green onions and sauté them lightly over medium heat until they are soft.
3. Stir in the refried beans. Cook until the beans are soft, stirring frequently.
4. Stir in the water until blended.
5. Stir in the salsa until blended.
6. Stir in the cheese until it has melted completely.
7. Remove the pan from the heat and spoon the dip into a serving bowl. Serve this dip with gluten-free tortilla chips.

*Makes 12 (¼-cup) servings*

One serving—Calories: 62; Total fat: 2.6 g; Saturated fat: 0.4 g; Cholesterol: 1 mg;
Sodium: 238 mg; Carbohydrates: 7.3 g; Fiber: 2 g; Sugar: 0.4 g; Protein: 2.6 g

# Almost Cheeseburger

½ pound lean ground beef

1 teaspoon dried onion flakes

1 pound shredded cheddar cheese
   (Vegan Gourmet Cheddar
   Cheese Alternative is dairy-free)

¼ cup milk (use casein-free soy or
   rice milk for dairy-free diets)

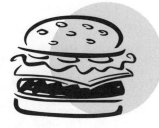

1 tablespoon ketchup (Heinz ketchup is gluten-free and dairy-free)

2 tablespoons yellow mustard

1. Spray a skillet with nonstick spray. Brown the beef and onion flakes in the skillet over medium-high heat, breaking up the meat with a fork as it cooks.
2. Lower the heat and stir in the cheese, milk, ketchup, and mustard. Continue stirring until the cheese has melted. Serve with gluten-free, dairy-free crackers or strips of bread.

*Makes 8 (½-cup) servings*

One serving—Calories: 123; Total fat: 4.8 g; Saturated fat: 1.2 g; Cholesterol: 33 mg; Sodium: 257 mg; Carbohydrates: 6 g; Fiber: 0.2 g; Sugar: 0.6 g; Protein: 13.5 g

## Homemade Peanut Butter

1 cup dry-roasted, unsalted peanuts

1 tablespoon peanut oil

1 teaspoon sugar

1. Put the nuts into a blender.
2. Put the lid on the blender and grind the nuts until they are very fine.
3. Add the oil and blend well, stopping to scrape the sides of the blender frequently with a rubber spatula.
4. Add the sugar and blend again until the mixture looks like peanut butter.

**Note:** If you like crunchy peanut butter, mix some finely chopped peanuts into your peanut butter.

*Makes about 12 (1-tablespoon) servings*

One serving—Calories: 79; Total fat: 7 g; Saturated fat: 1 g; Cholesterol: 0 mg; Sodium: 1.3 mg; Carbohydrates: 3.5 g; Fiber: 1 g; Sugar: 0.3 g; Protein: 2 g

# Trail Mix

4 cups Rice Chex Cereal (General Mills Rice Chex Cereal is now
   gluten-free)

¾ cup raisins

⅓ cup dried cranberries

½ cup dry-roasted peanuts

¼ cup sunflower seeds

½ cup coconut flakes

1 cup pretzels (Glutino makes gluten-free pretzels)

½ cup dried banana chips

1. Stir all of the ingredients together in a large bowl until evenly
   mixed.
2. Store the mix in a large self-seal plastic bag.

*Makes 16 (½-cup) servings*

One serving—Calories: 118; Total fat: 4.9 g; Saturated fat: 1.2 g; Cholesterol: 0 mg;
Sodium: 77 mg; Carbohydrates: 18.1 g; Fiber: 1.5 g; Sugar: 7.9 g; Protein: 2.4 g

# Homemade Granola

2 cups pure oats (Cream Hill Estates processes pure oats)

¾ cup slivered almonds

½ cup flaked, unsweetened coconut

½ cup cashews

⅓ cup brown sugar

1½ teaspoons allspice

1 teaspoon cinnamon

¼ cup butter (use dairy-free margarine for dairy-free diets)

3 tablespoons honey

1 cup pitted dates, each cut into thirds

1. Preheat oven to 300°F.
2. In a large bowl, mix together the oats, almonds, coconut,
   cashews, brown sugar, allspice, and cinnamon.

3. In a small saucepan, melt the butter or margarine with the honey over low heat.
4. Pour the butter-honey mixture over the granola mixture and toss well to coat all ingredients evenly.
5. Spread the mixture on a cookie sheet and bake for 20 minutes, stirring occasionally.
6. Add the dates, and mix to separate any clumps.
7. Continue to bake about 15 minutes more, stirring frequently, until the granola is golden brown.

**Note:** When the mixture has cooled, it will hold 2 weeks in an airtight container.

*Makes 12 (½-cup) servings*

One serving—Calories: 505; Total fat: 12.3 g; Saturated fat: 3.2 g; Cholesterol: 10.2 mg; Sodium: 33 mg; Carbohydrates: 33.5 g; Fiber: 6.6 g; Sugar: 19 g; Protein: 5.2 g

## Athena's Crunchy Pumpkin Seeds

This recipe was submitted by my 9½-year-old granddaughter!

2 cups pumpkin seeds fresh from a large pumpkin
1 teaspoon vanilla
¼ cup sugar
½ teaspoon cinnamon

1. Preheat oven to 350°F.
2. Cut the top off the pumpkin and scoop out the pulp that contains the seeds. Put the pulp in a colander and wash the pulp and stringy matter off the seeds under cold running water. Throw out the pulp, saving the seeds. Blot the seeds dry with paper towels.
3. Spread the seeds in a single layer on a cookie sheet. Sprinkle the seeds with the vanilla, then with the sugar and cinnamon.

④ Place the cookie sheet in the oven and bake the seeds for 10 minutes or until dry and lightly toasted. The cooking time will depend on the amount of seeds and how dry they were when they were put in the oven.

*Makes 16 (2-tablespoon) servings*

One serving—Calories: 113; Total fat: 7.9 g; Saturated fat: 1.5 g; Cholesterol: 0 mg; Sodium: 50 mg; Carbohydrates: 5 g; Fiber: 1 g; Sugar: 3.3 g; Protein: 4.2 g

## Caramel Popcorn

¼ cup butter (use dairy-free margarine for dairy-free diets; Fleischmann's makes a dairy-free margarine)

½ cup brown sugar

2 tablespoons light corn syrup

2 tablespoons honey

¼ teaspoon baking soda

4 cups popped popcorn

1 cup broken walnuts

① Put the butter, brown sugar, corn syrup, and honey in a large microwave-safe bowl. Microwave on high for 3 minutes and then stir the mixture.

② Add the baking soda. Stir carefully until the mixture is foamy.

③ Microwave the brown sugar sauce on high for another 1½ minutes.

④ Stir in the popcorn and walnuts until the popcorn is evenly coated with the sauce.

⑤ Microwave the popcorn mixture for 1 minute.

⑥ Spread the mixture onto a large sheet of wax paper. Let it cool at room temperature for 1 hour until it sets.

⑦ Break the mixture into pieces. Store in a gallon-size, reclosable plastic bag.

*Makes 11 (½-cup) servings*

One serving—Calories: 160; Total fat: 8.9 g; Saturated fat: 2.6 g; Cholesterol: 12 mg; Sodium: 62 mg; Carbohydrates: 19.8 g; Fiber: 1.1 g; Sugar: 14.2 g; Protein: 2 g

## Snack Puffs

½ cup butter (use dairy-free margarine for a dairy-free diet; Parkay margarine is dairy-free)

1 cup peanut butter

1½ cups chopped dark chocolate

1 (1-pound) box gluten-free, dairy-free puffed corn cereal (Arrowhead Mills makes a variety of gluten-free, dairy-free cereals)

1 (1-pound) box powdered sugar

1. Place the butter, peanut butter, and chocolate in a small microwave-safe bowl. Microwave on medium (50 percent power) for 1 minute.
2. Remove the bowl from the microwave, and stir the mixture.
3. Return the bowl to the microwave, and cook for 1 minute on medium. Stir, and continue the process of heating and stirring until the mixture is melted.
4. Place the cereal in a large bowl. Drizzle the chocolate mixture over the top to coat the cereal evenly.
5. Stir the cereal to distribute the chocolate coating evenly.
6. Empty the powdered sugar into a large paper bag and add the chocolate-coated cereal. Close the top of the bag securely.
7. Shake the bag until the sugar evenly coats the cereal mixture.

*Makes 24 (½-cup) servings*

One serving—Calories: 227; Total fat: 24 g; Saturated fat: 1.8 g; Cholesterol: 0.7 mg; Sodium: 41 mg; Carbohydrates: 23.1 g; Fiber: 2.3 g; Sugar: 15.7 g; Protein: 4.2 g

# Cereal Candy

3 cups gluten-free, dairy-free puffed rice cereal (Kallo Organic
    Puffed Rice Cereal is gluten- and dairy-free)

⅓ cup raisins

⅓ cup dried cranberries

⅓ cup dry-roasted peanuts

6 ounces dark chocolate, chopped into very small pieces

2 tablespoons light corn syrup

1. In a large bowl, stir together the cereal, raisins, cranberries, and peanuts.
2. Melt the chocolate in a medium glass bowl in the microwave, stirring every 30 seconds, until just melted.
3. Stir the corn syrup into the melted chocolate.
4. Carefully drizzle the melted chocolate mixture evenly over the cereal mix. Stir to mix.
5. Spoon the cereal candy into cupcake papers, then place the filled cups on a baking sheet.
6. Place the baking sheet in the refrigerator for 30 minutes to set the chocolate.

*Makes 10 (½-cup) servings*

One serving—Calories: 230; Total fat: 8.4 g; Saturated fat: 4.6 g; Cholesterol: 0 mg;
Sodium: 154 mg; Carbohydrates: 38 g; Fiber: 1.8 g; Sugar: 25.3 g; Protein: 3 g

# Rock Candy

2 cups + 2 cups sugar

1 cup water

¼ teaspoon blue food coloring (or your favorite color)

**You'll Need**

Glass jar

String

Pencil

Wax paper

1. In a medium saucepan, heat 2 cups of the sugar with the water. Stir until the sugar is completely dissolved.
2. Add the food coloring, and then slowly stir in the remaining 2 cups sugar, stirring constantly until the sugar is dissolved.
3. Carefully pour the mixture into a clean, quart-size glass jar. (You may want to use a funnel for this.)
4. Cut eight pieces of string, each 6 inches long. Tie one end of each string to the pencil.
5. Lay the pencil across the top of the jar so that the free ends of the strings hang into the sugar water. Lay a piece of wax paper over the top of the jar.
6. After a couple of hours, you will see crystals starting to form on the strings. The longer you leave the strings in the water, the thicker the crystals will get. Pieces can be broken off and eaten, then return the string to the sugar water to start building crystals again. The crystals will continue to build for several days or up to a week.

*Makes 8 (1-strand) servings*

One serving (after several days of accumulating crystals)   Calories: 339, Total fat: 0 g; Saturated fat: 0 g; Cholesterol: 0 mg; Sodium: 0 mg; Carbohydrates: 87.5 g; Fiber: 0 g; Sugar: 87.4 g; Protein: 0 g

## Chocolate Candy

You may want to substitute the raisins or nuts with ¼ cup of any of the following additional food items: coconut; pitted chopped dates; dried cranberries or dried cherries; chopped walnuts, pecans, or cashews; or 1 tablespoon raspberry preserves.

½ pound dark chocolate, chopped into small pieces

¼ teaspoon vanilla

⅓ cup raisins

⅓ cup plain salted peanuts or cashews

1. Put the chocolate in a 2-quart glass bowl.
2. Microwave on high for about 1½ minutes, stirring every 30 seconds, until just melted (do not overcook).
3. Remove the bowl from the microwave. Stir the chocolate until smooth.
4. If the chocolate has not melted, return the bowl to the microwave, and continue to cook on high until shiny. Be careful not to overcook or the chocolate could burn.
5. Remove the bowl from the microwave and stir the chocolate again until smooth. Stir in the vanilla.
6. Stir in the raisins and nuts.
7. Drop the candy by teaspoonfuls onto a cookie sheet. Refrigerate about 20 minutes or until firm.

*Makes 20 pieces*

One piece—Calories: 82; Total fat: 4.8 g; Saturated fat: 1.2 g; Cholesterol: 0.6 mg; Sodium: 15 mg; Carbohydrates: 9.26 g; Fiber: 1 g; Sugar: 6.8 g; Protein: 1.1 g

## Cranberry Candy

1 (15-ounce) can cranberry sauce

1 cup + 3 tablespoons granulated sugar

1 (3-ounce) box raspberry gelatin

1 (3-ounce) box lemon gelatin

½ cup finely chopped almonds

3 tablespoons powdered sugar

¼ teaspoon cinnamon

1. In a medium saucepan, stir together the cranberry sauce, 1 cup of granulated sugar, and the raspberry and lemon gelatins.
2. Bring the mixture to a boil over medium heat, stirring frequently. Remove the pan from the heat, and stir in the almonds.

3 Pour the mixture into a 9-inch square pan. Let the mixture cool, and then put it in the refrigerator for at least 6 hours.

4 Cut the gelled mixture into 1-inch squares.

5 Sift 3 tablespoons of granulated sugar, the powdered sugar, and the cinnamon together onto a piece of wax paper. Holding both sides of the wax paper, pour the sugar mixture into a gallon-size, self-seal plastic bag.

6 Place six squares of gelatin into the bag. (An easy way to loosen the gelled squares from the pan is to run a rubber spatula underneath them.) Seal the bag, and shake to coat all sides with sugar. Remove the squares, and arrange them on a plate. Repeat with the remaining squares, working in small batches.

7 When all the squares are coated with the sugar mixture, return them to the plastic bag. Seal it securely until ready to serve.

*Makes 81 (1-piece) servings*

One serving—Calories: 34; Total fat: 0.5 g; Saturated fat: 0 g; Cholesterol: 0 mg; Sodium: 12 mg; Carbohydrates: 7.5 g; Fiber: 0.2 g; Sugar: 7.2 g; Protein: 0.4 g

## Peanut Butter Cups

1½ cups chopped dark chocolate

½ cup creamy peanut butter

1 Line twelve mini-muffin tins with mini-muffin paper liners.

2 Put the chocolate pieces in a medium glass bowl and microwave for 1 minute, stirring the chocolate every 15 seconds until melted.

3 Spoon 1 tablespoon melted chocolate into each muffin paper liner.

4 Spoon 2 teaspoons peanut butter over the chocolate in each of the paper liners.

⑤ Spoon 1 tablespoon melted chocolate over the peanut butter in each of the paper liners.

⑥ Refrigerate the peanut butter cups for 2 hours or until they have hardened.

*Makes 12 servings*

One serving—Calories: 164; Total fat: 12.2 g; Saturated fat: 5.6 g; Cholesterol: 1 mg; Sodium: 58 mg; Carbohydrates: 16.2 g; Fiber: 2.3 g; Sugar: 12.8 g; Protein: 3.8 g

## Tortilla Snack

½ teaspoon butter (use dairy-free margarine for dairy-free diets)

1 gluten-free flour tortilla or corn tortilla (Mission corn tortillas are gluten-free)

½ teaspoon cinnamon sugar (or ½ teaspoon sugar mixed with ¼ teaspoon cinnamon)

① Preheat oven to 350°F.

② Spread the butter on one side of the tortilla. Sprinkle the cinnamon sugar on top.

③ Place tortilla in a small baking pan and bake for 4 minutes.

*Makes 1 serving*

One serving (made with a rice flour tortilla)—Calories: 140; Total fat: 2.4 g; Saturated fat: 1.2 g; Cholesterol: 5 mg; Sodium: 174 mg; Carbohydrates: 26.4 g; Fiber: 2.2 g; Sugar: 2.1 g; Protein: 0.01 g

## Fun Roll-Up

1 tablespoon peanut butter

1 gluten-free flour tortilla (Don Pancho makes gluten-free flour tortillas)

½ small banana, sliced

2 tablespoons chopped dark chocolate

1. Preheat oven to 350°F.
2. Spread the peanut butter evenly over the tortilla.
3. Lay the banana slices on one-half of the tortilla.
4. Sprinkle the chocolate over the banana slices.
5. Starting on the side with the bananas and chocolate, roll up the tortilla tightly.
6. Lay the tortilla on a piece of foil or in a small pan and bake for 4 minutes or until the chocolate has melted and the tortilla is lightly toasted.

*Makes 1 serving*

One serving—Calories: 421; Total fat: 19.6 g; Saturated fat: 7 g; Cholesterol: 1 mg; Sodium: 165 mg; Carbohydrates: 55.2 g; Fiber: 6.1 g; Sugar: 20.7 g; Protein: 6.1 g

## Rice Cake Bonanza

1 teaspoon peanut butter

1 gluten-free rice cake

1 teaspoon jelly (your favorite flavor)

1 teaspoon raisins

½ banana

2 marshmallows (most brands of marshmallows are dairy-free; AllerEnergy is one example)

1. Spread the peanut butter on one side of the rice cake.
2. Spread the jelly on top of the peanut butter.
3. Sprinkle the raisins on top of the jelly.
4. Slice the banana over the raisins, then top with the marshmallows.

*Makes 1 serving*

One serving—Calories: 191; Total fat: 3.2 g; Saturated fat: 1.7 g; Cholesterol: 0 mg; Sodium: 59 mg; Carbohydrates: 39.8 g; Fiber: 3 g; Sugar: 21.7 g; Protein: 3.3 g

# Creamy Pops

½ cup cranberry juice

1 cup milk (use casein-free vanilla soy milk or sweetened almond
   milk for dairy-free diets)

3 tablespoons sugar

1. In a medium bowl, stir together the juice, milk, and sugar.

2. Spoon the mixture into four Popsicle molds, or use 5-ounce paper cups.

3. Freeze the molds for 4 hours or until frozen solid. If you're using paper cups, insert a flat, wooden stick in the center of the mold when the mixture is partially frozen, then freeze until solid.

*Makes 4 pops*

One pop—Calories: 77; Total fat: 0.04 g; Saturated fat: 0 g; Cholesterol: 3 mg;
Sodium: 29 mg; Carbohydrates: 16.2 g; Fiber: 0.03 g; Sugar: 15.4 g; Protein: 1.6 g

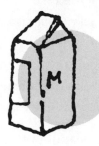

# 2
# Drinks

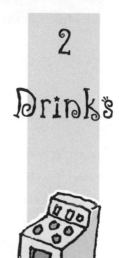

## Lime Fizz

Use your imagination to combine different flavors of soda and sorbet. Try orange sorbet with orange soda, or lemon sorbet with cherry soda.

¾ cup cold Sprite

¼ cup lime sorbet (use dairy-free sorbet for a dairy-free diet)

1. Pour half of the soda into a drinking glass.
2. Spoon the sorbet into the glass.
3. Pour in the remaining Sprite.

*Makes 1 (1-cup) serving*

One serving—Calories: 123; Total fat: 0 g; Saturated fat: 0 g; Cholesterol: 0 mg; Sodium: 21 mg; Carbohydrates: 33 g; Fiber: 0 g; Sugar: 11 g; Protein: 0 g

## Mint Lemon Fizz

2 cups cold water

⅔ cup fresh lemon juice (juice from 2 lemons)

⅓ cup sugar

4 fresh mint leaves

4 cups cold Sprite

Ice cubes

1 Pour the water into a large pitcher.

2 Pour the lemon juice through a strainer into the pitcher.

3 Stir in the sugar until completely dissolved.

4 Stir in the mint leaves.

5 Leave the pitcher on the counter for 30 minutes to let the flavors blend.

6 Remove the mint leaves.

7 Pour in the Sprite.

8 Put some ice cubes into each glass; pour the drink over the ice.

*Makes 7 (1-cup) servings*

One serving—Calories: 98; Total fat: 0 g; Saturated fat: 0 g; Cholesterol: 0 mg; Sodium: 13 mg; Carbohydrates: 26.3 g; Fiber: 0.09 g; Sugar: 10 g; Protein: 0.09 g

## Cherry Banana Shake

½ cup milk (use casein-free vanilla soy or rice milk for a dairy-free diet)

½ teaspoon vanilla

1 small ripe banana, sliced

6 maraschino cherries

1 tablespoon unsweetened cocoa

3 cups vanilla ice cream (Turtle Mountain makes dairy-free ice creams)

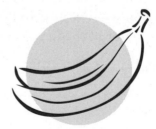

1 Put the milk (or vanilla soy or rice milk), vanilla, banana, cherries, and cocoa in a blender.

2 Cover and blend on high power until smooth.

3 Add the ice cream. Blend on medium power until smooth. Serve immediately.

*Makes 8 (½-cup) servings*

One serving—Calories: 155; Total fat: 6.5 g; Saturated fat: 3.6 g; Cholesterol: 22 mg; Sodium: 23 mg; Carbohydrates: 27.4 g; Fiber: 5.2 g; Sugar: 17.2 g; Protein: 1.5 g

## Chocolate Banana Whirl

½ cup milk (use casein-free vanilla soy milk or coconut milk for a dairy-free diet)

2 tablespoons grated dark chocolate

1 teaspoon vanilla

½ medium banana, sliced

1 Put the milk, chocolate, vanilla, and banana in a blender.

2 Blend on high until smooth. Pour into a glass.

*Makes 1 (1-cup) serving*

One serving—Calories: 226; Total fat: 9.4 g; Saturated fat: 6.1 g; Cholesterol: 5 mg; Sodium: 71 mg; Carbohydrates: 34.1 g; Fiber: 1.8 g; Sugar: 25.1 g; Protein: 5.8 g

## Peanut Butter Smoothie

¾ cup creamy peanut butter

¼ cup grated dark chocolate

1 teaspoon honey

1 cup milk (use casein-free vanilla soy milk or coconut milk for a dairy-free diet)

8 ice cubes

1 Put the peanut butter, chocolate, honey, milk, and ice in a blender.

2 Blend on high until smooth. Pour into three glasses.

*Makes 3 (1-cup) servings*

One serving—Calories: 560; Total fat: 38.7 g; Saturated fat: 10.8 g; Cholesterol: 7 mg; Sodium: 343 mg; Carbohydrates: 27.9 g; Fiber: 5 g; Sugar: 19 g; Protein: 19.6 g

# Apple Smoothie

1 apple, peeled, cored, and cut into chunks

1 small banana

⅓ cup milk (use casein-free vanilla soy or rice milk for a dairy-free diet)

⅛ teaspoon cinnamon

3 ice cubes

1 Put the apple, banana, milk, cinnamon, and ice cubes into a blender.

2 Blend on high until smooth, then pour into a glass.

*Makes 1 (1-cup) serving*

One serving—Calories: 208; Total fat: 2.2 g; Saturated fat: 1.1 g; Cholesterol: 7 mg; Sodium: 43 mg; Carbohydrates: 47.9 g; Fiber: 4.9 g; Sugar: 32.3 g; Protein: 4.2 g

# Peach Slush

½ cup milk (use casein-free vanilla soy milk or coconut milk for a dairy-free diet)

1 cup canned, juice-packed sliced peaches, drained

1 teaspoon sugar

¼ teaspoon vanilla

1 Pour the milk into an ice cube tray. If you don't have an ice cube tray, pour the milk into a shallow pan. Freeze for 1½ hours or until solid.

2 Put the peaches, sugar, and vanilla into a blender. Add the frozen cubes of milk. If the milk was frozen in a shallow pan, use a spoon or fork to break it up into smaller chunks before adding it to the blender.

3 Blend on high until smooth. Pour into three glasses.

*Makes 3 (½-cup) servings*

One serving—Calories: 63; Total fat: 0.9 g; Saturated fat: 0.5 g; Cholesterol: 3 mg; Sodium: 24 mg; Carbohydrates: 13 g; Fiber: 1.1 g; Sugar: 11.8 g; Protein: 1.9 g

# Raspberry Cooler

> 1 cup orange juice
>
> 1 cup frozen raspberries
>
> 1 tablespoon powdered sugar
>
> 1 cup crushed ice

1. Put the orange juice, raspberries, powdered sugar, and ice in a blender.
2. Blend on low speed until smooth. Pour into three glasses.

*Makes 3 (1-cup) servings*

One serving—Calories: 133; Total fat: 0.2 g; Saturated fat: 0.02 g; Cholesterol: 0 mg; Sodium: 1 mg; Carbohydrates: 32.9 g; Fiber: 3.8 g; Sugar: 20.7 g; Protein: 1.2 g

# Pineapple Berry Cooler

> 1 cup fresh strawberries, halved
>
> 1 cup pineapple chunks, fresh or canned
>
> ½ cup raspberries
>
> 3 tablespoons frozen lemonade concentrate, thawed
>
> Ice cubes

1. Wash the berries, remove the stems, and cut each strawberry in half.
2. Put the strawberries, pineapple, raspberries, and lemonade concentrate in a blender.
3. Blend on high until the mixture is smooth.
4. Put a few ice cubes into two glasses then pour in the berry cooler.

*Makes 2 (1-cup) servings*

One serving—Calories: 125; Total fat: 0.6 g; Saturated fat: 0.01 g; Cholesterol: 0 mg; Sodium: 2 mg; Carbohydrates: 31.8 g; Fiber: 4.6 g; Sugar: 24 g; Protein: 1.4 g

## Pineberry Drink

Ice cubes

¼ cup chilled pineapple juice

¼ cup chilled orange juice

¼ cup chilled cranberry juice

1 Put a few ice cubes into an 8-ounce glass.

2 Pour the pineapple, orange, and cranberry juices into the glass. Stir to blend.

*Makes 1 (¾-cup) serving*

One serving—Calories: 89; Total fat: 0.2 g; Saturated fat: 0.02 g; Cholesterol: 0 mg; Sodium: 3 mg; Carbohydrates: 22.1 g; Fiber: 0.3 g; Sugar: 13.9 g; Protein: 1 g

## Apricotberry Drink

1 (15-ounce) can juice-packed apricot halves, undrained

1 (10-ounce) package frozen raspberries

3 tablespoons honey

1 Put the apricot halves with their juice, the frozen raspberries, and honey in a blender.

2 Blend on medium speed until smooth.

*Makes 4 (¾-cup) servings*

One serving—Calories: 150; Total fat: 0.1 g; Saturated fat: 0 g; Cholesterol: 0 mg; Sodium: 4 mg; Carbohydrates: 39.1 g; Fiber: 4.1 g; Sugar: 34.9 g; Protein: 0.9 g

# Cranberry Punch

4 cups cranberry juice

1½ cups sugar

4 cups pineapple juice

1 cup orange juice

1 tablespoon almond extract

2 quarts Sprite

1. Combine the cranberry juice, sugar, pineapple juice, orange juice, and almond extract in a 1½-gallon pitcher. Stir until the sugar is dissolved.
2. Put the pitcher in the refrigerator for 2 hours to chill.
3. Pour the juice mixture into a punch bowl. Add the Sprite just before serving. Add ice to keep the punch cold.

*Makes 17 (1-cup) servings*

One serving—Calories: 156; Total fat: 0.2 g; Saturated fat: 0.02 g; Cholesterol: 0 mg; Sodium: 8 mg; Carbohydrates: 1.4 g; Fiber: 0.2 g; Sugar: 30.7 g; Protein: 0.6 g

# Cinnamon Hot Chocolate

2 tablespoons dark chocolate
   (approximately 2 squares from a
   6.8-ounce bar)

1 (3-inch) cinnamon stick

1 cup milk (use casein-free vanilla
   soy milk or almond milk for a
   dairy-free diet)

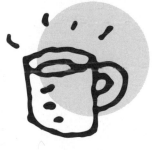

1. Using a grater, shave the chocolate. (Be careful not to scrape your fingers against the grater.)
2. Put the chocolate and cinnamon stick in a heatproof mug.

③ Pour the milk into a small saucepan and heat it on the stove just to a simmer. Do not let it boil.

④ Pour the hot milk into the mug. Stir until the chocolate has melted.

*Makes 1 (1-cup) serving*

One serving—Calories: 221; Total fat: 11.7 g; Saturated fat: 7.5 g; Cholesterol: 20 mg; Sodium: 133 mg; Carbohydrates: 26 g; Fiber: 1.7 g; Sugar: 22.8 g; Protein: 9.1 g

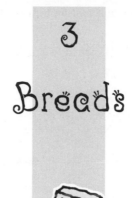

# Breads

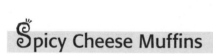

## Spicy Cheese Muffins

1 cup gluten-free flour mixture (See the Gluten-Free Flour Mixtures
   on page 16)

¼ teaspoon salt

5 teaspoons baking powder

¼ teaspoon garlic powder

⅓ cup sugar

3 tablespoons grated Parmesan cheese (Eat in the Raw Parma!
   Vegan Parmesan is dairy-free)

1½ teaspoons dried dill

1 egg

3 tablespoons milk (use casein-free soy or rice milk for dairy-free
   diets)

3 tablespoons vegetable oil

¼ cup salsa

¼ cup grated cheddar cheese (Vegan Gourmet Cheddar Cheese
   Alternative is dairy-free)

1 Preheat oven to 400°F. Spray 12 muffin cups with nonstick spray.

2 Put the flour mixture, salt, baking powder, garlic powder, sugar, Parmesan cheese, and dill into a medium bowl and whisk to blend.

3 In a small bowl, whisk together the egg, milk, and oil. Stir in the salsa.

4 Make a hole in the middle of the dry ingredients. Pour in the egg mixture. Add the cheddar cheese, then stir into the dry ingredients until evenly moistened.

5 Spoon the batter into the muffin cups, filling the cups three-quarters full.

6 Bake for 20 minutes or until a toothpick inserted in the center of the muffins comes out clean.

*Makes 12 muffins*

One muffin—Calories: 125; Total fat: 5.3 g; Saturated fat: 1.2 g; Cholesterol: 20 mg; Sodium: 334 mg; Carbohydrates: 17.4 g; Fiber: 0.6 g; Sugar: 7.5 g; Protein: 1.7 g

## Berry Delicious Muffins

⅔ cup dried cranberries

1½ cups fresh blueberries

⅓ cup + 2 tablespoons vegetable oil

1 tablespoon mayonnaise

2 eggs

1 teaspoon vanilla

1 teaspoon almond flavoring

1 tablespoon lemon juice

½ cup + 2 tablespoons milk (use casein-free vanilla soy milk or
    sweetened almond milk for dairy-free diets)

1¼ cups granulated sugar

½ teaspoon salt

¾ teaspoon + ½ teaspoon cinnamon

5 teaspoons baking powder

1 teaspoon baking soda

2 cups + 2 tablespoons gluten-free flour mixture (See the Gluten-
   Free Flour Mixtures on page 16)

½ cup slivered almonds, finely chopped

2 tablespoons brown sugar

½ teaspoon molasses

1. Preheat oven to 350°F. Spray muffin tins with nonstick spray.
2. Put the dried cranberries in a small bowl and cover with water, then set the bowl aside.
3. Put the blueberries in a strainer and wash them off under cold, running water. Set the strainer over a bowl to drain the berries. Set the bowl and strainer aside.
4. In a large bowl, using a wire whisk, mix the ⅓ cup oil, mayonnaise, eggs, vanilla, almond flavoring, lemon juice, and ½ cup milk together.
5. Stir the granulated sugar into the milk mixture.
6. Add the salt, ¾ teaspoon cinnamon, baking powder, baking soda, and 2 cups of the flour mixture and stir with a rubber spatula until the ingredients are blended.
7. Add the blueberries to the dough.
8. Drain the cranberries in the strainer, then add them to the dough.
9. Use the rubber spatula to fold in the berries.
10. Spoon the batter into the muffin tins, filling the tins two-thirds full.
11. In a small bowl, stir together 2 tablespoons oil, 2 tablespoons milk, 2 tablespoons flour mixture, chopped almonds, brown sugar, ½ teaspoon cinnamon, and molasses. Let set for 1 minute to thicken slightly. Spoon this mixture over the tops of the muffins, dividing evenly.
12. Bake the muffins 25 to 30 minutes or until a toothpick inserted in the center of the muffins comes out dry. Cool for 10 minutes before removing the muffins from the tins.

**Note:** These muffins are delicious soon after being baked, but they tend to dry out quickly. Freeze any muffins that will not be eaten the day they are baked. To defrost them, wrap them in a damp paper towel and heat in the microwave.

*Makes 20 muffins*

One muffin—Calories: 212; Total fat: 8.1 g; Saturated fat: 0.9 g; Cholesterol: 22 mg; Sodium: 230 mg; Carbohydrates: 33.6 g; Fiber: 1.6 g; Sugar: 18.4 g; Protein: 1.9 g

## Orange Muffins

⅓ cup orange juice

2 tablespoons orange zest

¼ cup applesauce

⅓ cup vegetable oil

2 teaspoons mayonnaise

2 teaspoons vanilla

2 eggs

½ cup brown sugar

2 cups gluten-free flour mixture (See the Gluten-Free Flour
     Mixtures on page 16)

2 tablespoons baking powder

¾ teaspoon cinnamon

½ teaspoon salt

1. Preheat oven to 350°F. Spray muffin tins with nonstick spray.
2. In a large bowl, whisk together the orange juice, zest, applesauce, oil, mayonnaise, vanilla, and eggs until well blended.
3. Stir in the brown sugar.
4. Add the flour mixture, baking powder, cinnamon, and salt. Stir just until all ingredients are completely blended.
5. Spoon the batter into the muffin tins.
6. Bake for 20 minutes or until a toothpick inserted in the center of the muffins comes out dry.

7 Let the muffins cool for 10 minutes before removing them from the muffin tins.

**Note:** Orange zest is grated orange peel. Grate the outside of the orange on a grater but don't grate so deeply into the skin that you grate the bitter white layer inside.

*Makes 12 muffins*

One muffin—Calories: 191; Total fat: 7.4 g; Saturated fat: 0.8 g; Cholesterol: 35 mg; Sodium: 290 mg; Carbohydrates: 29.9 g; Fiber: 1 g; Sugar: 9.1 g; Protein: 1.3 g

# Peanut Butter and Jelly Muffins

2 eggs

⅔ cup milk (use casein-free vanilla soy milk or sweetened almond milk for dairy-free diets)

2 teaspoons vanilla

3 tablespoons vegetable oil

½ cup sugar

1½ cups gluten-free flour mixture (See the Gluten-Free Flour Mixtures on page 16)

1 tablespoon baking powder

2 teaspoons baking soda

½ teaspoon salt

3 tablespoons peanut butter

3 tablespoons jelly or jam (your favorite flavor)

1 Preheat oven to 375°F. Spray muffin tins with nonstick spray.

2 Break the eggs into a large bowl and whisk until frothy. Add the milk, vanilla, and oil. Whisk until ingredients are blended.

3 Add the sugar and whisk again to blend.

4 Add the flour mixture, baking powder, baking soda, and salt. Stir with a rubber spatula until the mixture is smooth.

⑤ Fill each of 18 muffin tins one-third full with batter. Spoon ½ teaspoon peanut butter onto the center of the batter. Spoon ½ teaspoon jelly or jam on top of the peanut butter. Spoon batter over the peanut butter and jelly, covering them completely, until each tin is three-quarters full.

⑥ Bake for 20 minutes or until a toothpick inserted in the center of a muffin comes out clean. Remove the muffins from the tins and let them cool on a wire rack.

*Makes 18 muffins*

One muffin—Calories: 122; Total fat: 4.6 g; Saturated fat: 0.8 g; Cholesterol: 24 mg; Sodium: 290 mg; Carbohydrates: 18.3 g; Fiber: 0.7 g; Sugar: 8 g; Protein: 2 g

## Pineapple Coconut Muffins

1 egg

⅔ cup vanilla ice cream, softened (use dairy-free ice cream for dairy-free diets; Turtle Mountain makes dairy-free ice cream)

⅔ cup sugar

6 tablespoons pineapple preserves

1 tablespoon vegetable oil

2 teaspoons vanilla

1 tablespoon mayonnaise

1 cup gluten-free flour mixture (See the Gluten-Free Flour Mixtures on page 16)

2 teaspoons baking powder

1¼ teaspoons baking soda

¼ teaspoon salt

¼ cup shredded coconut

① Preheat oven to 350°F. Spray 12 muffin tins with nonstick spray.

② In a large bowl, whisk the egg slightly.

③ Whisk in the ice cream, sugar, preserves, oil, vanilla, and mayonnaise.

④ With a rubber spatula, stir in the flour mixture, baking powder, baking soda, and salt.

⑤ Stir in the coconut.

⑥ Fill each muffin tin about two-thirds full with batter.

⑦ Bake for 20 minutes or until a toothpick inserted in the center of a muffin comes out clean.

*Makes 12 muffins*

One muffin—Calories: 156; Total fat: 10 g; Saturated fat: 1.2 g; Cholesterol: 21 mg; Sodium: 269 mg; Carbohydrates: 37 g; Fiber: 0.8 g; Sugar: 18.2 g; Protein: 1.2 g

## Peanut Butter Banana Muffins

1 egg

¼ cup mashed banana (about 1 banana mashed with a fork)

2 tablespoons peanut butter

1 teaspoon vanilla

1½ tablespoons vegetable oil

2 tablespoons milk (use casein-free soy milk or almond milk for dairy-free diets)

¼ cup granulated sugar

¼ cup brown sugar

¼ teaspoon salt

1¼ cups gluten-free flour mixture (See the Gluten-Free Flour Mixtures on page 16)

1 tablespoon baking powder

1 teaspoon baking soda

½ cup chopped dark chocolate

① Preheat oven to 350°F. Spray 12 muffin tins with nonstick spray.

② Break the egg into a large bowl. Whip with a wire whisk until frothy.

③ Add the banana, peanut butter, vanilla, oil, and milk and whisk until smooth.

④ Whisk in the granulated and brown sugars.

⑤ Add the salt, flour mixture, baking powder, and baking soda. Use a rubber spatula to blend all the ingredients.

⑥ Stir in the chocolate.

⑦ Spoon the batter into the muffin tins, filling each about two-thirds full. Bake for 20 minutes or until a toothpick inserted in the center of the muffin comes out clean.

*Makes 12 muffins*

One muffin—Calories: 161; Total fat: 5.9 g; Saturated fat: 2.1 g; Cholesterol: 18 mg; Sodium: 268 mg; Carbohydrates: 36.8 g; Fiber: 1.4 g; Sugar: 13.6 g; Protein: 2.2 g

## Harvest Muffins

1 cup chopped pitted dates

½ cup raisins

¾ cup water

2 eggs, slightly beaten

½ cup brown sugar

½ cup unsweetened applesauce

¼ cup orange juice

¼ cup olive oil

2 teaspoons vanilla

1½ teaspoons almond extract

½ cup chopped nuts

2 cups gluten-free flour mixture (See the Gluten-Free Flour Mixtures on page 16)

¼ teaspoon salt

2 teaspoons baking soda

1 tablespoon baking powder

¾ teaspoon cinnamon

① Preheat oven to 350°F. Spray muffin tins with nonstick spray.

② Put the dates and raisins in a large saucepan. Add the water, and bring to a boil on the stove. Boil until the water has been absorbed (about 4 minutes). Remove the pan from the heat and let mixture cool.

3  In large bowl, beat the eggs with a fork until frothy. Stir in the brown sugar, applesauce, orange juice, olive oil, vanilla, and almond extract.

4  Stir the dates and raisins into the egg mixture. Stir in the nuts.

5  Add the flour mixture, salt, baking soda, baking powder, and cinnamon and stir with a rubber spatula just until the ingredients are blended.

6  Spoon the batter into the muffin tins, filling each muffin cup two-thirds full.

7  Bake for 15 minutes or until a toothpick inserted in the center of a muffin comes out clean.

8  Remove the hot tins from the oven. Let the muffins sit for 10 minutes before removing them from the muffin tins.

**Note:** An easy way to "chop" dates is to cut them with wet scissors.

*Makes 18 muffins*

One muffin  Calories: 174; Total fat: 6 g; Saturated fat: 0.6 g; Cholesterol: 23 mg; Sodium: 243 mg; Carbohydrates: 29.3 g; Fiber: 2 g; Sugar: 14.4 g; Protein: 2.1 g

## Carrot Muffins

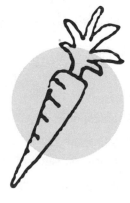

1 egg
¼ cup vegetable oil
2 teaspoons vanilla
1 teaspoon almond flavoring
½ cup granulated sugar
½ cup brown sugar
1½ cups grated carrots
¼ cup crushed pineapple, undrained
2½ teaspoons baking powder

2 teaspoons baking soda

¼ teaspoon salt

½ teaspoon cinnamon

1¾ cups gluten-free flour mixture (See the Gluten-Free Flour Mixtures on page 16)

¾ cup raisins

½ cup chopped walnuts

1. Preheat oven to 350°F. Spray 24 muffin tins with nonstick spray.
2. In a large bowl, use a whisk to whip the egg until frothy.
3. Whisk in the oil, vanilla, almond flavoring, granulated sugar, and brown sugar.
4. Using a rubber spatula, stir in the carrots and crushed pineapple.
5. Add the baking powder, baking soda, salt, cinnamon, and flour mixture. Stir till blended.
6. Stir in the raisins and walnuts.
7. Spoon the batter into the muffin tins. Bake for 18 minutes or until a toothpick inserted in the center of the muffins comes out clean.

*Makes 24 muffins*

One muffin—Calories: 127; Total fat: 4.3 g; Saturated fat: 0.4 g; Cholesterol: 9 mg; Sodium: 177 mg; Carbohydrates: 21.8 g; Fiber: 1 g; Sugar: 12.1 g; Protein: 1.2 g

## Corn Muffins

1¼ cups milk (use casein-free soy or rice milk for dairy-free diets)

1 teaspoon cider vinegar

1 egg

3 tablespoons olive oil

¾ cup sugar

½ teaspoon salt

1 cup cornmeal

1¼ cups gluten-free flour mixture (See the Gluten-Free Flour
  Mixtures on page 16)
1½ tablespoons baking powder
1½ teaspoons baking soda

1. Preheat oven to 400°F. Spray 20 muffin tins with nonstick spray.
2. In a small bowl, stir together the milk and vinegar. Let it set for 5 minutes. (The milk may look a little lumpy, but that's OK.)
3. Whip the egg in a large bowl with a wire whisk until frothy. Add the milk mixture, oil, and sugar and whip till blended.
4. Stir in the salt, cornmeal, flour mixture, baking powder, and baking soda until completely blended.
5. Spoon the mixture into the muffin cups, filling each cup two-thirds full.
6. Bake for 18 to 20 minutes or until a toothpick inserted in the center comes out clean.

**Note:** I recommend that you use a fine-ground yellow cornmeal for this recipe. It is worth buying a high-grade cornmeal because it will definitely enhance the taste of these muffins.

*Makes 20 muffins*

One muffin—Calories: 112; Total fat: 3.1 g; Saturated fat: 0.7 g; Cholesterol: 12 mg; Sodium: 246 mg; Carbohydrates: 19.9 g; Fiber: 0.8 g; Sugar: 8.4 g; Protein: 1.6 g

## Lemon Raspberry Muffins

1 egg
¾ cup milk
⅓ cup vegetable oil
1½ teaspoons lemon extract
1 teaspoon vanilla
¾ cup sugar

1½ cups gluten-free flour mixture (See the Gluten-Free Flour
Mixtures on page 16)

2 tablespoons baking powder

½ teaspoon salt

1 cup fresh raspberries, washed and drained

1 Preheat oven to 375°F. Spray 12 muffin tins with nonstick
spray.

2 Break the egg into a medium bowl and whip with a wire whisk
until frothy.

3 Add the milk, oil, lemon extract, vanilla, and sugar. Whisk
until mixture is smooth.

4 Add the flour mixture, baking powder, and salt and stir with
a rubber spatula until smooth.

5 Very carefully fold in the raspberries.

6 Spoon the batter into the muffin tins, filling each tin two-
thirds full. Bake for 20 minutes or until a toothpick inserted
in the center comes out clean.

*Makes 12 muffins*

One muffin—Calories: 185; Total fat: 7.3 g; Saturated fat: 0.9 g; Cholesterol: 19 mg:
Sodium: 291 mg; Carbohydrates: 28.6 g; Fiber: 1.4 g; Sugar: 13.9 g; Protein: 1.7 g

## Apple Bread

2 eggs

⅓ cup vegetable oil

¼ cup applesauce

2½ teaspoons vanilla

1¼ cups brown sugar

1 cup peeled, cored, and grated apple

½ cup chopped walnuts

1 teaspoon grated orange zest

1¾ cups gluten-free flour mixture (See the Gluten-Free Flour
Mixtures on page 16)

1 tablespoon baking soda

2 teaspoons baking powder

¼ teaspoon salt

2¼ teaspoons cinnamon

½ teaspoon nutmeg

1 Preheat oven to 350°F. Spray four 3″ × 5″ mini loaf pans with nonstick spray.

2 In a large bowl, whisk the eggs until frothy.

3 Add the oil, applesauce, vanilla, and brown sugar and whisk until blended.

4 Stir in the apples, walnuts, and orange zest.

5 Add the flour mixture, baking soda, baking powder, salt, cinnamon, and nutmeg. Stir with a rubber spatula until completely blended.

6 Pour the batter into the four pans. Bake for 35 minutes or until a toothpick inserted in the center comes out clean.

7 Remove the pan from the oven and let it set for 10 minutes, then turn the pan upside down to remove the loaf. Let the loaf cool, right side up, on a wire rack.

**Note:** Orange zest is grated orange peel. Grate the outside of the orange, being careful not to grate into the bitter white layer under the peel.

*Makes 4 mini loaves*

One loaf—Calories: 542; Total fat: 31.2 g; Saturated fat: 3.2 g; Cholesterol: 106 mg; Sodium: 1,328 mg; Carbohydrates: 125.5 g; Fiber: 5.2 g; Sugar: 72.6 g; Protein: 7.6 g

# Pumpkin Bread

1¼ cups dried cranberries

3 eggs

2 cups canned pumpkin

3 tablespoons molasses

⅓ cup vegetable oil

⅓ cup applesauce

2 teaspoons vanilla

1 teaspoon almond flavoring

¾ cup granulated sugar

¾ cup brown sugar

3¾ cups gluten-free flour mixture
   (See the Gluten-Free Flour
   Mixtures on page 16)

1 tablespoon baking powder

2 teaspoons baking soda

¾ teaspoon salt

2 teaspoons cinnamon

½ teaspoon nutmeg

½ teaspoon ground cloves

¾ cup chopped pecans

1. Preheat oven to 325°F. Spray eight 3″ × 5½″ mini loaf pans with nonstick spray.

2. Put the cranberries in a small bowl and cover with water. Set bowl aside.

3. Break the eggs into a separate large bowl and whisk until foamy.

4. Whisk in the pumpkin, molasses, oil, applesauce, vanilla, almond flavoring, granulated sugar, and brown sugar.

5. Add the flour mixture, baking powder, baking soda, salt, cinnamon, nutmeg, and cloves. Stir with a rubber spatula until the mixture is well blended.

6. Drain the cranberries in a sieve. Stir cranberries and pecans into the batter.

7. Spoon the batter into the mini baking pans. Bake for 30 minutes or until a toothpick inserted in the center of the breads comes out clean.

**Note:** The reason mini loaf pans are used instead of one large baking pan is that they bake much more evenly and thoroughly when baked in smaller pans.

*Makes 8 mini loaves*

One loaf—Calories: 663; Total fat: 19.5 g; Saturated fat: 2.1 g; Cholesterol: 79 mg; Sodium: 854 mg; Carbohydrates: 119.7 g; Fiber: 7 g; Sugar: 58.8 g; Protein: 6.1 g

## Soft Cheese Pretzels

For a birthday party, you can make pretzels in the shape of your age or the letters of your name!

¼ teaspoon + ¼ teaspoon salt

2 tablespoons + 1½ teaspoons sugar

½ teaspoon dried dill

2¾ tablespoons dry yeast

1½ teaspoons baking powder

1½ cups gluten-free flour mixture (See the Gluten-Free Flour Mixtures on page 16)

⅔ cup warm (not hot) water

¾ cup grated cheddar cheese (Vegan Gourmet Cheddar Cheese Alternative is dairy-free)

1 egg, beaten

1. Preheat oven to 425°F. Lightly spray a baking sheet with nonstick spray.
2. In a large bowl, use a whisk to blend together ¼ teaspoon salt, sugar, dill, yeast, baking powder, and flour mixture.
3. With a rubber spatula, stir in the warm water until blended. Stir in the cheese.
4. Sprinkle your hands with a little flour mixture, and then knead the dough to blend in the cheese.
5. Divide the dough into 18 balls (about the size of Ping-Pong balls).

6. Rub your hands with a little flour mixture. On a lightly floured board, roll each ball into a rope shape about 10 inches long, and then fold the rope into a pretzel shape. Place the pretzels on the baking sheet.

7. In a small bowl, beat the egg using a fork or whisk. Brush the tops of the pretzels with the beaten egg, and sprinkle the tops of the pretzels with the remaining ¼ teaspoon salt.

8. Bake for 15 minutes.

*Makes 18 pretzels*

One pretzel—Calories: 71; Total fat: 2 g; Saturated fat: 1.1 g; Cholesterol: 17 mg; Sodium: 96 mg; Carbohydrates: 11.1 g; Fiber: 0.6 g; Sugar: 1.8 g; Protein: 2 g

## Sesame Crackers

1 cup sesame seeds

2 cups gluten-free flour mixture (See the Gluten-Free Flour
  Mixtures on page 16)

½ teaspoon salt

1 teaspoon dried dill

½ teaspoon garlic powder

¼ cup brown sugar

⅓ cup olive oil

¼ cup applesauce

1 egg white

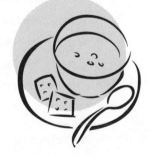

1. Preheat oven to 425°F. Spray a baking sheet with nonstick spray.

2. Put the sesame seeds in a pie plate that has been sprayed with nonstick spray. Toast the seeds in the hot oven for about 4 minutes or just until the seeds start to brown. Watch them closely so they don't burn. Remove the pie plate from the oven and let the seeds cool.

3. Lower the oven temperature to 375°F.

④ Put the flour mixture, salt, dill, garlic powder, and brown sugar into a medium mixing bowl. Use a rubber spatula to stir in the oil and applesauce until all is moistened.

⑤ Add the sesame seeds, mixing them in thoroughly.

⑥ Place the dough on a sheet of wax paper. Cover the dough with a second sheet of wax paper. Using a rolling pin, roll out the dough to ¼-inch thickness.

⑦ Remove the top sheet of wax paper. Cut the rolled dough into 1½″ × 2″ rectangles. Place the rectangles on the baking sheet. Reroll any leftover dough and cut into rectangles.

⑧ In a small bowl, whisk together the egg white with 2 tablespoons of water. Use a pastry brush to brush this mixture on top of the crackers.

⑨ Poke the top of each cracker in two different places with a fork.

⑩ Put the baking sheet in the oven and bake for 10 to 12 minutes or until the edges just begin to brown. Do not overbake the crackers or they will become too hard. Remove the baking sheet from the oven and let the crackers cool.

*Makes 50 crackers*

One cracker—Calories: 53; Total fat: 2.9 g; Saturated fat: 0.4 g; Cholesterol: 0 mg; Sodium: 25 mg; Carbohydrates: 6.3 g; Fiber: 0.6 g; Sugar: 1.2 g; Protein: 0.8 g

# Personal Pan Pizza Crust

½ cup gluten-free flour mixture (See the Gluten-Free Flour Mixtures on page 16)

1 tablespoon fine-ground cornmeal

1½ teaspoons baking powder

⅛ teaspoon salt

½ teaspoon garlic powder

½ teaspoon Italian seasoning

1 teaspoon grated Parmesan cheese (Eat in the Raw Parma! Vegan Parmesan is dairy-free)

1 tablespoon olive oil

⅓ cup milk (use casein-free soy or rice milk for dairy-free diets)

1. Preheat oven to 425°F. Spray a baking sheet with nonstick spray.

2. In a medium bowl, use a whisk to mix the flour mixture, cornmeal, baking powder, salt, garlic powder, Italian seasoning, and Parmesan cheese together.

3. Use a rubber spatula to stir in the oil and milk.

4. Spray two sheets of wax paper on one side with nonstick spray. Form the dough into a ball and place it on the sprayed side of one sheet of wax paper. Top with the other sheet of wax paper, sprayed side down. Use a rolling pin to roll the dough into a 9-inch circle.

5. Remove the top sheet of wax paper. Transfer the dough circle to the baking sheet.

6. Crimp the edges of the dough to form a raised edge.

7. Bake the crust for 5 minutes. Do not overbake or the pizza crust may become too hard. Remove the pan from the oven and top with your favorite toppings. Return the pan to the oven for 5 more minutes.

*Makes 1 personal pan pizza crust*

One crust—Calories: 497; Total fat: 17.6 g; Saturated fat: 3.7 g; Cholesterol: 8 mg; Sodium: 895 mg; Carbohydrates: 75.4 g; Fiber: 4.1 g; Sugar: 5.2 g; Protein: 7.2 g

# 4

# Breakfasts

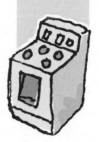

## Layered Breakfast Casserole

1 (10-ounce) bag frozen hash brown potatoes

1 cup cooked ham, cut into ½-inch cubes (use casein-free ham for
a dairy-free diet)

¼ cup thinly sliced green onions

6 eggs

1 cup milk (use casein-free soy or rice milk for a dairy-free diet)

½ teaspoon dry mustard

¼ teaspoon salt

¼ teaspoon pepper

1½ cups grated cheddar cheese (Vegan Gourmet Cheddar Cheese
Alternative is dairy-free)

1 large tomato

1 Preheat oven to 350°F. Spray a 9-inch square baking dish with
nonstick spray.

2 Line the bottom of the baking dish with the hash brown potatoes. Sprinkle the ham cubes on top of the potatoes. Sprinkle
the onions over the ham.

3. In a medium bowl, whisk together the eggs, milk, dry mustard, salt, and pepper. Pour the egg mixture over the ham.

4. Sprinkle the grated cheese on top of the egg mixture.

5. Cut the tomato into thin slices. Lay the slices on top of the cheese.

6. Bake for 45 to 50 minutes or until firm.

*Makes 6 (3" × 4½") servings*

One serving—Calories: 284; Total fat: 17.3 g; Saturated fat: 8.7 g; Cholesterol: 256 mg; Sodium: 702 mg; Carbohydrates: 13.4 g; Fiber: 1.2 g; Sugar: 4.6 g; Protein: 19.5 g

## Breakfast Quiche

1 (10-ounce) box frozen chopped broccoli, thawed and
   squeezed dry

1 small onion, chopped

¾ cup grated cheddar cheese (Vegan Gourmet Cheddar Cheese
   Alternative is dairy-free)

¼ cup + ¼ cup grated Monterey Jack cheese (Vegan Gourmet
   Monterey Jack Cheese Alternative is
   dairy-free)

4 eggs

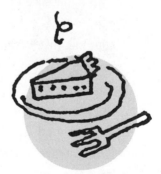

1½ cups milk (use casein-free soy or
   rice milk for dairy-free diets)

½ teaspoon salt

¼ teaspoon pepper

¼ teaspoon dried dill

3 tablespoons cornstarch

1. Preheat oven to 350°F. Spray a 9-inch pie plate with nonstick spray.

2. Place the broccoli in the bottom of the pie plate. Sprinkle the onion on top of the broccoli. Sprinkle the cheddar cheese and ¼ cup of the Monterey Jack cheese on top of the onion.

3 Put the eggs, milk, salt, pepper, dill, and cornstarch into a blender. Blend on high for 1 minute.

4 Pour the egg mixture over the cheese in the pie plate. Sprinkle remaining ¼ cup Monterey Jack cheese on top.

5 Bake for 40 minutes or until a knife inserted in the center comes out clean. Let the quiche rest for 5 minutes before cutting it into wedges.

*Makes 6 wedges*

One wedge—Calories: 173; Total fat: 10.3 g; Saturated fat: 5.2 g; Cholesterol: 162 mg; Sodium: 389 mg; Carbohydrates: 9.6 g; Fiber: 1.5 g; Sugar: 4.2 g; Protein: 11.3 g

## Breakfast Enchiladas

4 gluten-free corn tortillas (Taco Del Mar makes gluten-free corn tortillas)

4 slices gluten-free deli ham (use casein-free ham for a dairy-free diet)

1¼ cups grated cheddar cheese (Vegan Gourmet Cheddar Cheese Alternative is dairy-free)

¼ cup chopped green onion

½ cup chopped green pepper

3 eggs

1 cup milk (use casein-free soy or rice milk for a dairy-free diet)

¼ cup salsa

2 teaspoons cornstarch

⅛ teaspoon salt

⅛ teaspoon black pepper

⅛ teaspoon red pepper flakes

1 Preheat oven to 350°F. Spray a 9-inch square baking dish with nonstick spray.

2 Wrap the tortillas in foil. Bake for 5 minutes to soften them.

3 Lay out the tortillas. Lay one slice of ham on each tortilla. Sprinkle one-quarter of the cheese on each tortilla.

④ Place one-quarter of the onion and green pepper pieces on each tortilla.

⑤ Roll up each tortilla and place it, seam side down, in the dish.

⑥ In a medium bowl, mix the eggs, milk, salsa, cornstarch, salt, black pepper, and red pepper flakes with a fork. Pour the egg mixture over the tortillas.

⑦ Spray one side of a 12-inch square piece of foil with nonstick spray. Cover the baking dish with the foil, sprayed side down.

⑧ Bake for 35 minutes, then remove the foil and continue to bake for another 10 minutes.

*Makes 4 (1-enchilada) servings*

One serving—Calories: 468; Total fat: 21.4 g; Saturated fat: 10.3 g; Cholesterol: 218 mg; Sodium: 862 mg; Carbohydrates: 45.8 g; Fiber: 4.3 g; Sugar: 5 g; Protein: 21 g

## Farmer's Eggs

1 (14½-ounce) can potatoes, drained

½ pound sausage (Uncured Natural Meats has gluten-free, dairy-free sausage)

½ green pepper, diced

8 eggs

⅛ teaspoon salt

⅛ teaspoon black pepper

¼ cup salsa

① Cut the potatoes into small chunks; set aside.

② In a large skillet, cook the sausage and green pepper, breaking up the meat with a fork, until the sausage is browned.

③ Add the potatoes and cook for 1 more minute, stirring often.

④ Break the eggs into a medium bowl. Add the salt and black pepper and whisk until very frothy.

⑤ Add the eggs to the sausage and cook, stirring constantly, until the eggs are no longer wet. Stir in the salsa.

*Makes 6 servings*

One serving—Calories: 252; Total fat: 17.2 g; Saturated fat: 5.4 g; Cholesterol: 313 mg; Sodium: 580 mg; Carbohydrates: 7.8 g; Fiber: 1.4 g; Sugar: 1.7 g; Protein: 8.6 g

## Ham and Egg Cups

4 medium slices deli ham (use casein-free ham for a dairy-free diet)

1 small tomato

4 eggs

Dash salt

Dash pepper

① Preheat oven to 350°F.

② Spray four custard cups with nonstick spray. Put a round slice of ham in the bottom and up the sides of each cup.

③ Cut the tomato into four slices. Place one tomato slice on top of each piece of ham. Break an egg into each cup. Sprinkle lightly with salt and pepper.

④ Bake for 15 minutes or until the egg is cooked the way you like it.

*Makes 4 (1-cup) servings*

One serving—Calories: 107; Total fat: 6.1 g; Saturated fat: 2 g; Cholesterol: 226 mg; Sodium: 467 mg; Carbohydrates: 1.7 g; Fiber: 0.3 g; Sugar: 1.4 g; Protein: 11.4 g

## Breakfast in a Mug

This can be assembled ahead, covered, and refrigerated. In the morning, pop it into the microwave. Cook a little longer if it has been refrigerated.

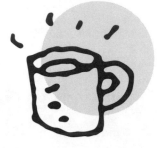

1 egg

3 tablespoons milk (use casein-free soy or rice milk for dairy-free diets)

1 small dash gluten-free Worcestershire sauce (Lea & Perrins Worcestershire Sauce is gluten- and dairy-free in the United States; the Canadian version has malt added and is not gluten-free)

¼ teaspoon dry mustard

Dash of pepper

1 slice gluten-free bread, cut into ¼-inch cubes (use dairy-free bread for dairy-free diets; Ener-G Foods Papa's Bread is gluten- and dairy-free)

¼ cup cooked ham, cut into small cubes

2 tablespoons shredded cheddar cheese (Vegan Gourmet Cheddar Cheese Alternative is dairy-free)

1 Spray a mug with nonstick spray.

2 In a small bowl, whisk the egg until frothy. Add the milk, Worcestershire sauce, dry mustard, and pepper; continue to whisk until blended.

3 Stir in the bread cubes, ham, and cheese.

4 Pour the mixture into the mug. Cover the mug with a large piece of wax paper and tuck the wax paper under the mug. With a knife, cut one slit in the top of the wax paper to vent.

5 Place the mug in the microwave and cook on medium-high (80 percent power) for 4½ minutes or until the mixture is just set.

*Makes 1 serving*

One serving—Calories: 254; Total fat: 13.2 g; Saturated fat: 5.8 g; Cholesterol: 246 mg; Sodium: 624 mg; Carbohydrates: 15.2 g; Fiber: 1.4 g; Sugar: 4.7 g; Protein: 18.8 g

## PB&J Toasted Sandwiches

5 eggs

1¼ cups milk (use casein-free vanilla soy or rice milk for a dairy-free diet)

3 tablespoons sugar

1 tablespoon vanilla

4 tablespoons peanut butter

8 slices gluten-free bread (Tapioca Loaf from Ener-G Foods is gluten- and dairy-free)

4 tablespoons jelly (your favorite flavor)

1 large banana

2 teaspoons vegetable oil

1 In a shallow bowl, whisk the eggs slightly. Add the milk, sugar, and vanilla. Whisk again until all ingredients are well blended.

2 Spread 1 tablespoon of peanut butter on each of four slices of bread. Spread 1 tablespoon jelly over the peanut butter on the four slices of bread.

3 Cut the banana into 16 slices. Lay four banana slices on top of the jelly on each of the four slices of bread. Put the four remaining slices of bread on top of the banana layers to form four sandwiches.

4 Preheat a large, nonstick skillet or griddle on the stove for 1 minute. Spray the pan with nonstick spray or lightly brush the pan with the oil.

5 Soak one sandwich at a time in the egg mixture, carefully turning it over one time, until both sides are covered with the egg mixture.

6) Working in batches if necessary, place the soaked sandwiches in the skillet or on the griddle. Cook the sandwiches, turning them once with a spatula, until they are golden on both sides.

*Makes 4 (1-sandwich) servings*

One serving—Calories: 509; Total fat: 21.5 g; Saturated fat: 4 g; Cholesterol: 272 mg; Sodium: 364 mg; Carbohydrates: 60.9 g; Fiber: 4.6 g; Sugar: 31.6 g; Protein: 19.5 g

## Night-Before Breakfast Sandwiches

1¼ cups milk (use casein-free soy or rice milk for dairy-free diets)

4 eggs

¾ teaspoon vanilla

½ teaspoon cinnamon

¼ teaspoon salt

8 slices gluten-free bread
   (use dairy-free bread for
   dairy-free diets)

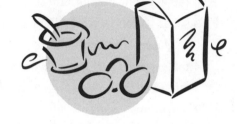

4 slices American cheese
   (Vegan Gourmet Cheddar Cheese Alternative is dairy-free)

4 thin slices ham (use casein-free ham for dairy-free diets)

½ cup gluten-free cornflakes (use dairy-free cornflakes for dairy-free diets; Honey'd Corn Flakes Cereal from Nature's Path is gluten- and dairy-free)

2 tablespoons butter (use dairy-free margarine for dairy-free diets)

1) In a medium bowl, whisk together the milk, eggs, vanilla, cinnamon, and salt.

2) Generously spray a 9-inch square pan with gluten-free nonstick spray. Pour a third of the egg mixture into the bottom of the pan.

3) Cut the crusts from the bread and discard. Place four slices of bread in the pan.

4) Lay one slice of cheese and one slice of ham on each piece of bread in the pan. Top with the four remaining bread slices. Pour the remaining egg mixture over the bread in the pan.

5. Cover with plastic wrap. Refrigerate for at least 8 hours (so the bread absorbs the moisture).

6. Preheat oven to 350°F.

7. Put the cornflakes in a plastic bag, and crush them with a rolling pin. Transfer the crumbs to a small bowl. Melt the butter in a glass measuring cup in the microwave. Pour the melted butter over the cornflakes, and mix to blend. Sprinkle the cereal mixture over the top of the casserole.

8. Bake uncovered for 40 minutes. If desired, serve with maple syrup.

*Makes 4 (4½-inch square) servings*

One serving—Calories: 400; Total fat: 20.3 g; Saturated fat: 9.6 g; Cholesterol: 258 mg; Sodium: 1,030 mg; Carbohydrates: 33.6 g; Fiber: 3 g; Sugar: 7.8 g; Protein: 21.71 g

## Mashed Breakfast

This is also good spread on untoasted gluten-free bread to pack for a school lunch.

    1 small ripe banana, peeled
    1 tablespoon peanut butter
    2 teaspoons jelly
    1 slice gluten-free bread (use dairy-free bread for dairy-free diets;
        Kinnikinnick Tapioca Rice Bread is gluten- and dairy-free)

1. Cut the banana into several chunks. Put the banana in a sandwich-size, reclosable plastic bag. Add the peanut butter and the jelly to the bag.

2. Seal the bag securely. Have fun smushing, mashing, and rolling the contents of the bag until they are well blended.

3. Toast the bread in the toaster. Spread your "banana mash" on the toast.

*Makes 1 serving*

One serving—Calories: 287; Total fat: 9.6 g; Saturated fat: 1 g; Cholesterol: 0 mg; Sodium: 126 mg; Carbohydrates: 47 g; Fiber: 5 g; Sugar: 21.5 g; Protein: 7.6 g

# Night-Before Oven French Toast

Serve French toast dusted with powdered sugar or topped with maple syrup, pancake syrup, jelly, fresh strawberries, or blueberries. Or sprinkle with toasted almonds.

> 6 eggs
>
> 3 tablespoons sugar
>
> 1 teaspoon cinnamon
>
> 1 cup milk (use casein-free vanilla soy or almond milk for a
>     dairy-free diet)
>
> 1 teaspoon vanilla
>
> ¼ teaspoon almond extract
>
> 8 slices gluten-free, dairy-free bread (Gillian's makes gluten- and
>     dairy-free bread)

1. Spray a cookie sheet with nonstick spray.
2. Break the eggs into a wide bowl. Add the sugar, cinnamon, milk, vanilla, and almond extract. Use a wire whisk to beat the mixture until it is well blended.
3. Dip each bread slice into the mixture, and then turn the bread over so all sides are covered with the egg mixture. Place the bread on the cookie sheet.
4. After all the bread slices have been dipped, pour any remaining liquid evenly over them. Cover the cookie sheet with plastic wrap. Refrigerate the cookie sheet overnight, giving the bread time to absorb the liquid.
5. The next morning, preheat oven to 350°F.
6. Bake the French toast for 10 minutes and then carefully turn over the slices. Continue to bake the toast for an additional 10 to 15 minutes or until the toast is lightly browned.

*Makes 4 (2-slice) servings*

One serving—Calories: 325; Total fat: 13.4 g; Saturated fat: 3.5 g; Cholesterol: 353 mg; Sodium: 429 mg; Carbohydrates: 44.2 g; Fiber: 4.3 g; Sugar: 17.4 g; Protein: 13.4 g

# Banana Pancakes

For extra fun, add two small circles of batter near the top of each pancake to form the head of Mickey Mouse!

1 medium ripe banana

2 eggs

¾ teaspoon vanilla

1¼ cups milk (use casein-free vanilla soy milk or
    vanilla almond milk for a dairy-free diet)

1 tablespoon vegetable oil

¾ cup gluten-free flour mixture (See
    the Gluten-Free Flour Mixtures on
    page 16)

1 tablespoon sugar

¼ teaspoon cinnamon

1 teaspoon baking powder

¼ teaspoon salt

1. In a medium-size bowl, mash the banana with a fork.
2. Whisk the eggs, vanilla, milk, and oil into the banana until well mixed.
3. Add the flour mixture, sugar, cinnamon, baking powder, and salt to the egg mixture. Whisk the batter until smooth. Let mixture sit for 10 minutes.
4. Spray a large skillet or griddle with nonstick spray. Set the skillet or griddle on the stove to preheat. Using a ¼-cup measure or a small ladle, spoon the batter into the pan.
5. Cook the pancakes over medium heat until small bubbles appear on top. Gently turn the pancakes over, using a spatula, and let them cook till the bottoms are lightly browned.

*Makes 4 (3-pancake) servings*

One pancake—Calories: 81; Total fat: 2.9 g; Saturated fat: 0.8 g; Cholesterol: 38 mg; Sodium: 101 mg; Carbohydrates: 11.6 g; Fiber: 0.6 g; Sugar: 3.7 g; Protein: 2.2 g

## Cornmeal Pancakes

1 cup milk (use casein-free soy or rice milk for a dairy-free diet)

2 teaspoons lemon juice

3 eggs

¼ cup vegetable oil

1¼ cups gluten-free flour mixture
   (See the Gluten-Free Flour
   Mixtures on page 16)

2 tablespoons brown sugar

¾ cup cornmeal (use a fine-ground
   cornmeal)

2 teaspoons baking powder

1 teaspoon baking soda

¼ teaspoon salt

½ teaspoon cinnamon

Maple syrup

1  In a small bowl, stir together the milk and lemon juice. Set bowl aside for 5 minutes. (The mixture may look curdled, but it's supposed to.)

2  Put the eggs in a blender. Blend on high speed for 5 seconds. Add the milk and oil and blend for 10 seconds.

3  Add the flour mixture, brown sugar, cornmeal, baking powder, baking soda, salt, and cinnamon. Blend the batter for 1 minute, stopping the blender every 20 seconds to scrape the sides.

4  Spray a large skillet or griddle with nonstick spray. Preheat the pan or griddle on the stove. When the pan is hot, use a baster or ladle to spoon ½ cup of the batter into the pan.

5  When bubbles appear around the edges, turn the pancake over so it can brown on the other side. Repeat until you have used all the batter. Serve with maple syrup.

**Note:** It is recommended that you use a fine-ground yellow corn-meal for this recipe. It is worth buying a high-grade cornmeal because it will definitely enhance the taste of these pancakes.

*Makes 5 (2-pancake) servings*

One pancake (without maple syrup)—Calories: 200; Total fat: 8.2 g; Saturated fat: 1.4 g; Cholesterol: 66 mg; Sodium: 290 mg; Carbohydrates: 27.3 g; Fiber: 1.2 g; Sugar: 4.3 g; Protein: 4.1 g

## Microwave Oatmeal

⅓ cup pure oats (Cream Hill Estates processes pure oats)

⅔ cup water

¼ teaspoon cinnamon

1 tablespoon brown sugar

2 tablespoons raisins or dried cranberries

1 tablespoon chopped walnuts

¼ cup milk (use casein-free vanilla soy milk or almond milk for a dairy-free diet)

1. Place the oats and water in a microwave-safe bowl that can hold at least 2 cups. Microwave, uncovered, on high, until the oatmeal is thick and almost all the water has been absorbed (about 1½ to 2½ minutes).
2. Remove the bowl from the microwave. Stir in the cinnamon and brown sugar.
3. Let the oatmeal stand for about 1 minute to finish absorbing the water.
4. Stir in the raisins (or cranberries) and walnuts.
5. If you like thinner oatmeal, just before serving stir in some milk.

*Makes 1 serving*

One serving—Calories: 207; Total fat: 2 g; Saturated fat: 0 g; Cholesterol: 0 mg; Sodium: 11 mg; Carbohydrates: 46 g; Fiber: 4 g; Sugar: 19.8 g; Protein: 4 g

## Apple Rice Pudding

¼ cup maple syrup

1 tablespoon butter (use dairy-free margarine for those on a dairy-free diet; Earth Balance is gluten- and dairy-free)

¼ teaspoon cinnamon

⅛ teaspoon nutmeg

1 apple, peeled and chopped into small pieces

1 cup cooked brown rice

1 cup milk (use casein-free vanilla soy or almond milk for those on a dairy-free diet)

⅓ cup raisins

3 tablespoons slivered almonds

1 Heat the maple syrup, butter, cinnamon, nutmeg, and chopped apple in a skillet until the mixture is bubbling.

2 Stir in the rice, milk, raisins, and almonds. Simmer for about 10 minutes, stirring occasionally, until the mixture thickens. Serve in bowls.

*Makes 3 (¾-cup) servings*

One serving—Calories: 344; Total fat: 10.4 g; Saturated fat: 4.3 g; Cholesterol: 18 mg; Sodium: 69 mg; Carbohydrates: 57.5 g; Fiber: 3.2 g; Sugar: 35.7 g; Protein: 6.3 g

## Blueberry Coffee Cake

1 egg

3 tablespoons + 1 teaspoon orange juice

⅔ cup vanilla ice cream, softened (use dairy-free ice cream for dairy-free diets; Turtle Mountain makes dairy-free ice cream)

3 tablespoons vegetable oil

2 teaspoons vanilla

1 cup sugar

2 cups gluten-free flour mixture (See the Gluten-Free Flour Mixtures on page 16)

2 tablespoons baking powder

½ teaspoon salt

1 teaspoon cinnamon

1½ cups blueberries

**Topping**

3 tablespoons sugar

¼ teaspoon cinnamon

2 tablespoons chopped walnuts

1. Preheat oven to 350°F. Spray a 9-inch square baking pan with nonstick spray.
2. Break the egg into a large bowl. Add the orange juice, ice cream, oil, vanilla, and sugar. Mix well with a whisk.
3. Add the flour mixture, baking powder, salt, and cinnamon. Stir until just blended.
4. Spread the batter in the pan. Sprinkle the blueberries on top of the batter.
5. In a small bowl, stir together the topping ingredients: sugar, cinnamon, and chopped nuts. Sprinkle the mixture on top of the batter.
6. Bake for 35 minutes or until a toothpick inserted in the center of the coffee cake comes out clean.

*Makes 9 (3-inch square) servings*

One serving—Calories: 310; Total fat: 7.7 g; Saturated fat: 1.3 g; Cholesterol: 28 mg, Sodium: 388 mg; Carbohydrates: 58.4 g; Fiber: 2.2 g; Sugar: 31.2 g; Protein: 2.5 g

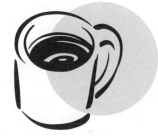

# 5
# Main Dishes

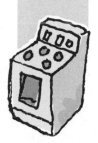

## Spaghetti Pie

1 tablespoon olive oil

½ pound uncooked gluten-free spaghetti

2 cups gluten-free, dairy-free spaghetti sauce (Prego Traditional
Italian Sauce is gluten- and diary-free)

½ cup + ½ cup grated mozzarella cheese (Vegan Gourmet
Mozzarella Cheese Alternative is dairy-free)

¼ teaspoon red pepper flakes

1 teaspoon Italian seasoning

¼ teaspoon garlic powder

1 tablespoon dried parsley flakes

1. Preheat oven to 350°F. Brush olive oil on the bottom and sides
of a 9-inch pie plate.

2. Break the dry spaghetti strands into thirds. Cook the spaghetti
in a large pot of boiling water as the package directs. Do not
overcook the pasta or it will become mushy. Once cooked,
very carefully pour the pasta and water in a colander so the
pasta can drain.

③ Put the spaghetti back into pan. Pour the spaghetti sauce over the spaghetti. Sprinkle ½ cup cheese, the red pepper flakes, Italian seasoning, garlic powder, and parsley over the spaghetti. Stir spaghetti with a fork to mix everything evenly.

④ Spoon the spaghetti into the pie plate. With the back of a spoon, smooth the top. Sprinkle the remaining ½ cup cheese on top.

⑤ Spray a 10-inch square piece of foil with nonstick spray. Cover the pie plate with the foil, sprayed side down. Put the pan in the oven and bake for 30 minutes. To serve, cut the pie into 6 wedges.

*Makes 6 (1-wedge) servings*

One serving (made with rice pasta)—Calories: 260; Total fat: 10.8 g; Saturated fat: 3.9 g; Cholesterol: 13 mg; Sodium: 808 mg; Carbohydrates: 32.1 g; Fiber: 5 g; Sugar: 15.3 g; Protein: 8.3 g

## Tuna Noodle Casserole

3 ounces gluten-free noodles

1 (6-ounce) can water-packed tuna fish, drained (do not use canned albacore tuna for dairy-free diets; StarKist Chunk Light Tuna in spring water is casein-free)

1 green onion, minced

¼ cup chopped celery

¼ cup chopped green pepper

⅓ cup frozen peas

⅓ cup shredded cheddar cheese (Vegan Gourmet Cheddar Cheese Alternative is dairy-free)

1 cup gluten-free chicken broth (Swanson Chicken Broth is gluten- and dairy-free)

¼ cup mayonnaise

¼ teaspoon black pepper

¼ teaspoon dried dill

¼ cup gluten-free bread crumbs (Nu-World Amaranth Bread
Crumbs are gluten- and dairy-free)

¼ cup chopped almonds

½ teaspoon paprika

1 tablespoon vegetable oil

1. Preheat oven to 350°F. Spray a 9-inch square baking dish with nonstick spray.

2. Fill a large pan two-thirds full with water and bring the water to a boil. Stir in the noodles and boil them until they are just tender (about 5 minutes). Drain the noodles in a colander and place them in a large bowl.

3. Stir in the tuna fish, green onion, celery, green pepper, peas, cheese, broth, mayonnaise, black pepper, and dill. Spoon the mixture into the baking dish.

4. In a small bowl, stir together the bread crumbs, almonds, and paprika. Add the oil and stir until everything is evenly moistened. Sprinkle the crumbs on top of the casserole.

5. Bake uncovered for 30 minutes or until contents are heated through.

*Makes 4 (2-cup) servings*

One serving—Calories: 350; Total fat: 17.2 g; Saturated fat: 3.6 g; Cholesterol: 26 mg; Sodium: 729 mg; Carbohydrates: 31 g; Fiber: 2.6 g; Sugar: 2.9 g; Protein: 18.2 g

# Tuna Puff

5 slices gluten-free bread, cut into ¼-inch cubes (Glutino White
Rice Bread is gluten- and dairy-free)

1 cup shredded cheddar cheese (Vegan Gourmet Cheddar Cheese
Alternative is dairy-free)

1 (12-ounce) can tuna fish, drained (do not use canned albacore
tuna for dairy-free diets; StarKist Chunk Light Tuna in spring
water is casein-free)

1 tablespoon dried minced onion

3 eggs

2 cups milk (use casein-free soy or rice milk for dairy-free diets)

½ teaspoon salt

⅛ teaspoon paprika

1 Preheat oven to 325°F. Spray an 8-inch square baking pan with nonstick spray.

2 Spread half of the bread cubes on the bottom of the baking pan. Sprinkle half of the cheese over the bread in the pan. Crumble the tuna over the cheese layer. Sprinkle the onion flakes over the tuna. Top with remaining bread cubes, then sprinkle with remaining cheese.

3 In a small bowl, whisk the eggs until frothy. Whisk in the milk and salt. Pour this over the cheese in the baking pan. Sprinkle the top lightly with paprika.

4 Bake for 45 minutes or until firm, or until a knife inserted in the center comes out clean.

**Note:** This dish is best when it's assembled early in the day, covered, and refrigerated for several hours so the bread has a chance to absorb part of the liquid.

*Makes 4 servings*

One serving—Calories: 418; Total fat: 26.3 g; Saturated fat: 9.9 g; Cholesterol: 224 mg; Sodium: 1,011 mg; Carbohydrates: 24.8 g; Fiber: 2.1 g; Sugar: 9.2 g; Protein: 39.5 g

## Tuna Melt

1 (6½-ounce) can water-packed tuna, drained (do not use canned albacore tuna for dairy-free diets; StarKist Chunk Light Tuna in spring water is casein-free)

1 rib celery, diced

2 tablespoons minced green pepper

1 green onion, minced

¼ cup mayonnaise

4 slices gluten-free, dairy-free bread (Glutino Rice Fiber Bread is
   gluten- and dairy-free)

4 thin slices tomato

¼ cup grated cheddar cheese (Vegan Gourmet Cheddar Cheese
   Alternative is dairy-free)

1 Preheat broiler.

2 In a small bowl, stir together the tuna, celery, green pepper,
   onion, and mayonnaise until well mixed.

3 Place the bread slices on a broiler pan.

4 With a knife, spread one-fourth of the tuna mixture on each
   piece of bread.

5 Place a slice of tomato on top of each sandwich.

6 Sprinkle one-fourth (1 tablespoon) of the
   cheese on top of each sandwich.

7 Broil the sandwiches about 3 minutes,
   or just until the tops begin to bubble
   and are golden.

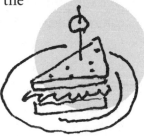

*Makes 4 sandwiches*

One sandwich—Calories: 205; Total fat: 8.8 g;
Saturated fat: 2.5 g; Cholesterol: 24 mg; Sodium: 291 mg; Carbohydrates: 16.4 g;
Fiber: 1.8 g; Sugar: 4 g; Protein: 12.7 g

## Tuna Stuffed Peppers

4 large cubanelle peppers, cut in half lengthwise and membrane
   removed

1 egg

½ cup milk (use casein-free soy or rice milk for dairy-free diets)

1 teaspoon lemon juice

¼ teaspoon salt

¼ teaspoon black pepper

2 tablespoons finely chopped onion

2 slices gluten-free bread (Ener-G Foods Brown Rice Bread is
   gluten- and dairy-free)

1 (12-ounce) can tuna fish, drained (do not use canned albacore tuna for dairy-free diets; StarKist Chunk Light Tuna in spring water is casein-free)

2 tablespoons gluten-free seasoned bread crumbs (Gillian's bread crumbs are gluten- and dairy-free)

1 Preheat oven to 400°F. Spray an 8½″ × 11″ baking pan with nonstick spray.

2 Put the cubanelle peppers in a medium saucepan, cover with water, and bring to a boil on the stove. Boil for 5 minutes. Drain, then run cold water over the peppers to cool them off. Drain again, then place peppers on paper toweling to remove remaining moisture.

3 In a medium bowl, whip the egg with a fork until frothy. Add the milk, lemon juice, salt, black pepper, and onion and whip again with a fork to blend. Crumble the bread slices into the egg mixture, and then stir in the tuna fish till blended.

4 With a spoon, fill the pepper shells with the tuna mixture, dividing mixture evenly. Place filled shells in the baking pan. Sprinkle each top with ½ tablespoon bread crumbs.

5 Bake for 15 minutes or until heated through.

*Makes 4 servings*

One serving—Calories: 195; Total fat: 4 g; Saturated fat: 1.3 g; Cholesterol: 78 mg; Sodium: 619 mg; Carbohydrates: 14.9 g; Fiber: 1.1 g; Sugar: 3 g; Protein: 24.2 g

## Cod Fish Sticks

½ cup milk (use casein-free soy or rice milk for dairy-free diets)

2 teaspoons lemon juice

1 pound cod, cut into 1″ × 3″ strips

½ cup gluten-free flour mixture (See the Gluten-Free Flour Mixtures on page 16)

½ teaspoon salt

½ teaspoon pepper

¼ teaspoon garlic powder

2 eggs

¼ cup cornmeal

⅓ cup gluten-free bread crumbs (use dairy-free bread crumbs for dairy-free diets)

⅓ cup gluten-free crushed puffed rice cereal (Nature's Path Organic Crispy Rice Cereal is gluten- and dairy-free)

¾ teaspoon paprika

1. Preheat oven to 425°F. Lightly spray a baking sheet with non-stick spray.
2. In a medium-size bowl, stir together the milk and lemon juice. Let it set for 5 minutes. (The mixture will look curdled.) Add the strips of cod and let them soak in the milk mixture while you get the remaining ingredients ready.
3. Put the flour mixture, salt, pepper, and garlic powder into a self-seal plastic bag. Use a spoon to mix the ingredients.
4. In a shallow bowl, whisk the eggs until they are frothy.
5. In another self-seal bag, stir together the cornmeal, bread crumbs, crushed cereal, and paprika.
6. Remove the cod from the milk and place the strips in the bag with the flour mixture. Seal the bag, then shake it well to coat the pieces of fish evenly with flour.
7. Remove the fish strips and place them in the egg mixture. Use your fingers or a spoon to cover each strip with the egg mixture.
8. Remove the strips from the egg mixture and place them in the bag with the cornmeal mixture. Seal the bag, then shake it well to coat the pieces of fish evenly.
9. Place the breaded pieces of fish on the baking sheet. Spray the tops of the fish with nonstick spray.
10. Bake for 10 minutes, then turn the pieces over and bake 10 minutes more or until the fish flakes easily with a fork.

*Makes 4 servings*

One serving—Calories: 292; Total fat: 5.2 g; Saturated fat: 1.7 g; Cholesterol: 157 mg; Sodium: 596 mg; Carbohydrates: 32.5 g; Fiber: 1.8 g; Sugar: 2.9 g; Protein: 27.1 g

# Maple Syrup Salmon

3 salmon fillets, 5 ounces each

⅓ cup maple syrup

2 teaspoons lemon juice

1 tablespoon gluten-free soy sauce
(San-J Organic Wheat Free
Tamari Soy Sauce is gluten- and
dairy-free)

⅛ teaspoon ground ginger

⅛ teaspoon pepper

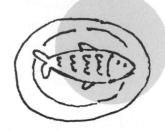

1. Preheat oven to 425°F. Spray a 9-inch square baking pan with nonstick spray.
2. Wash the salmon, then lay the damp salmon pieces in the baking dish, skin side down.
3. In a bowl, stir together the maple syrup, lemon juice, soy sauce, ginger, and pepper. Spoon this mixture over the salmon.
4. Bake salmon for 15 to 20 minutes or until it flakes easily when tested with a fork.

*Makes 3 servings*

One serving—Calories: 378; Total fat: 12.7 g; Saturated fat: 2 g; Cholesterol: 109 mg; Sodium: 426 mg; Carbohydrates: 24.4 g; Fiber: 0.05 g; Sugar: 21.3 g; Protein: 39.9 g

# Meat Loaf Muffins

1 cup gluten-free, dairy-free crushed puffed rice cereal (Erewhon
Crispy Brown Rice Cereal is gluten- and dairy-free)

½ cup warm water

1 pound lean ground beef

2 tablespoons dried parsley flakes

1 envelope dry onion soup mix (Connor Creek French Onion Soup
Mix is gluten- and dairy-free)

1 egg

2 tablespoons + 2 tablespoons ketchup (Heinz ketchup is gluten-
and dairy-free)

1 Preheat oven to 350°F. Spray 6 muffin tins with nonstick spray.

2 Put the crushed puffed rice into a medium bowl. Add the water and let the cereal soak for 1 minute to soften.

3 Add the ground beef, parsley, onion soup mix, egg, and 2 tablespoons ketchup.

4 With your hands (washed just before and afterward), blend the mixture well.

5 Divide the meat mixture into six portions; pack each portion into a muffin tin. Bake for 20 minutes.

6 Remove the tins from the oven. Spread the remaining 2 tablespoons ketchup evenly over the tops of the muffins. Return the tins to the oven, and bake 20 minutes more.

**Note:** An easy way to crush puffed rice cereal is to put it into a sandwich bag, seal the bag, then use a rolling pin to crush the contents.

*Makes 6 (1-muffin) servings*

One serving—Calories: 159; Total fat: 4.4 g; Saturated fat: 1.8 g; Cholesterol: 75 mg; Sodium: 721 mg; Carbohydrates: 11.1 g; Fiber: 0.7 g; Sugar: 3.1 g; Protein: 16.8 g

# Four-Ingredient Casserole

1 pound lean ground beef

1 (32-ounce) bag frozen hash brown potatoes, thawed

1 (26-ounce) jar gluten-free spaghetti sauce (Classico Roasted Garlic Pasta Sauce is gluten- and dairy-free)

1 cup + 1 cup shredded mozzarella cheese (Vegan Gourmet Mozzarella Cheese Alternative is dairy-free)

1. Preheat oven to 350°F. Spray a 9″ × 11″ pan with nonstick spray.
2. Put the beef in a microwave-safe shallow container and break the meat up with a fork. Microwave on high for 1 minute. Remove and break up the meat with a fork. Repeat this process until the meat is browned. Drain off any juices.
3. Layer half of the potatoes in the bottom of the pan. Top with half of the spaghetti sauce. Spread the cooked beef on top of the sauce. Sprinkle with 1 cup of the cheese. Spread remaining spaghetti sauce, then top with the remaining 1 cup cheese. Sprinkle the top with the remaining half of the potatoes.
4. Bake for 45 minutes.

*Makes 8 (1¾-cup) servings*

One serving—Calories: 338; Total fat: 12 g; Saturated fat: 5.8 g; Cholesterol: 52 mg; Sodium: 633 mg; Carbohydrates: 34.3 g; Fiber: 4.2 g; Sugar: 9.4 g; Protein: 22.5 g

## Taco Casserole

1 pound lean ground beef

1 medium onion, chopped

3 cups crushed gluten-free tortilla chips (Santitas white corn tortilla chips are gluten- and dairy-free)

1 (15½-ounce) jar medium-hot salsa

1 cup shredded cheddar cheese (Vegan Gourmet Cheddar Cheese Alternative is dairy-free)

1. Crumble the ground beef into a microwave-safe pan. Mix in the onion. Microwave the meat and onion on high, uncovered, for 2 minutes. Remove the pan, and break up the pieces of meat with a fork. Return the meat to the microwave and cook 2 minutes more, then again break up the meat into small pieces. If needed, repeat this process one more time until the meat is browned.
2. Put the meat and onion in a colander to drain off any fats that have accumulated.

③ Spray a 9-inch square microwave-safe casserole with nonstick spray.

④ Layer 1 cup of the tortilla chips in the bottom of the casserole. Spread the ground beef and onion mixture over the chips. Spoon the salsa over the meat layer.

⑤ Sprinkle the cheese, then the remaining tortilla chips over the top of the casserole.

⑥ Microwave the casserole on high, uncovered, for 3 minutes, then rotate the dish. Microwave for 3 more minutes or until the casserole is heated through. If more cooking time is needed, rotate the dish again before continuing. The casserole dish may be hot, so use a pot holder to rotate it and to remove it from the oven.

*Makes 6 (3" × 4½") servings*

One serving—Calories: 373; Total fat: 16.1 g; Saturated fat: 6.6 g; Cholesterol: 66 mg; Sodium: 1,012 mg; Carbohydrates: 32.1 g; Fiber: 2.3 g; Sugar: 7.6 g; Protein: 22.8 g

## Really Great Taco Salad

½ cup mayonnaise

¼ cup red taco sauce (mild or medium, depending on taste)

½ teaspoon lemon juice

½ teaspoon cider vinegar

½ head iceberg lettuce, chopped

2 tomatoes, chopped

1 small onion, chopped

½ green pepper, chopped

¼ cup pitted sliced black olives

1 small (6-ounce) can kidney beans, drained

8 ounces grated cheddar cheese (Vegan Gourmet Cheddar Cheese Alternative is gluten- and dairy-free)

¾ pound lean ground beef

1½ tablespoons gluten-free taco seasoning mix

4 cups gluten-free tortilla chips, broken into chunks

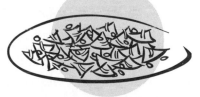

1 In a small bowl, stir together the mayonnaise, taco sauce, lemon juice, and vinegar. Set this salad dressing aside.

2 In a large bowl, toss together the lettuce, tomatoes, onion, green pepper, olives, beans, and cheese.

3 Place the beef in a microwave-safe baking pan, breaking it up into small chunks with a fork. Microwave on high for 2 minutes. Remove pan and continue to break up meat into smaller chunks with a fork. Microwave for another minute. Remove pan and use a spoon to remove and discard pan juices. Stir in the taco seasoning mix and microwave for 1 minute more.

4 Spoon the beef over the lettuce, add the tortilla chips and salad dressing, and toss well.

*Makes 4 (2-cup) servings*

One serving—Calories: 804; Total fat: 43.6 g; Saturated fat: 17.9 g; Cholesterol: 144 mg; Sodium: 1,496 mg; Carbohydrates: 56.9 g; Fiber: 6.9 g; Sugar: 8.3 g; Protein: 46.5 g

## Dinner in a Pouch

2 large potatoes

½ green pepper

1 medium onion

¼ teaspoon salt

¼ teaspoon black pepper

1 (15-ounce) can corn kernels, drained

½ cup water

1 (15½-ounce) jar salsa

1 pound lean ground beef

1 Preheat oven to 400°F.

2 Cut four 20″ × 18″ pieces of heavy-duty foil. Fold each in half to form an 18″ × 10″ rectangle.

3 Cut the potatoes into ½-inch cubes. Slice the green pepper and onion into thin slices.

4 In a large bowl, stir together the potatoes, green pepper, onion, salt, black pepper, corn, water, and salsa.

5 Divide the beef into four equal portions. Form a patty out of each portion. Place a beef patty in the center of each piece of foil.

6 Spoon one-fourth of the potato mixture over each beef patty.

7 Wrap each packet securely, using double-fold seals. (Allow some room for heat expansion.)

8 Place the packets on a cookie sheet. Bake for 1 hour.

*Makes 4 servings (¼ pound beef plus ½ potato and 4 ounces vegetables)*

One serving—Calories: 393; Total fat: 9.5 g; Saturated fat: 3.3 g; Cholesterol: 81 mg; Sodium: 1,194 mg; Carbohydrates: 41.3 g; Fiber: 3.3 g; Sugar: 11 g; Protein: 34.6 g

## Skillet Supper

1 pound lean ground beef

2 cups water

1 (15-ounce) jar spaghetti sauce (Classico Tomato and Basil Pasta Sauce is gluten- and dairy-free)

1 teaspoon oregano

2 cups gluten-free elbow macaroni

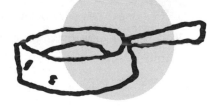

½ cup shredded mozzarella cheese (Vegan Gourmet Mozzarella Cheese Alternative is dairy-free)

¾ cup grated Parmesan cheese (Eat in the Raw Parma! Vegan Parmesan is dairy-free)

1 Brown the ground beef in a large skillet over medium-high heat, breaking up the meat with a fork. When the meat is browned, stir in the water, spaghetti sauce, and oregano. Bring to a simmer over medium heat.

2 Stir in the macaroni. Cover the pan, and simmer for 6 minutes until the macaroni is just cooked, stirring frequently. Stir in the cheeses. Cover the pan and let stand for 1 minute or until the cheese is melted.

*Makes 4 (2-cup) servings*

One serving—Calories: 849; Total fat: 19.9 g; Saturated fat: 9.5 g; Cholesterol: 124 mg; Sodium: 1,056 mg; Carbohydrates: 112.3 g; Fiber: 5 g; Sugar: 10.6 g; Protein: 49.1 g

## Love That Chili!

1 tablespoon olive oil

¾ pound lean ground beef

1 large onion, chopped

½ green pepper, chopped

1 (8-ounce) can tomato sauce

¼ cup water

1 (15-ounce) can light red kidney beans, undrained

1 (15-ounce) can navy beans, drained

½ teaspoon garlic powder

1¼ teaspoons chili powder

¼ teaspoon cayenne

1 teaspoon unsweetened cocoa

½ teaspoon sugar

½ teaspoon salt

¼ teaspoon black pepper

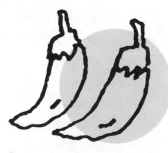

1 Heat the olive oil in a medium pot on the stove for 30 seconds over medium-high heat. Add the ground beef, onion, and

green pepper and cook, breaking up the meat with a fork, until the meat is browned.

2 Stir in the tomato sauce, water, kidney beans with their juice, navy beans, garlic powder, chili powder, cayenne, cocoa, sugar, salt, and black pepper.

3 Reduce the heat to a simmer. Cover the pot, and let the chili simmer slowly for 1 hour.

**Note:** You can also make this chili in a slow cooker. Brown the meat, onions, and green pepper on the stove, as in step 1. Transfer the mixture to a slow cooker. Stir in the remaining ingredients, as in step 2. Cover the pot and cook on low heat for 8 hours. If you like your chili really spicy, increase the amount of chili powder and cayenne. If you like it really mild, use a little less chili powder and cayenne than what is listed in the ingredients.

*Makes 4 (1-cup) servings*

One serving—Calories: 305; Total fat: 8.8 g; Saturated fat: 2.7 g; Cholesterol: 51 mg; Sodium: 1,153 mg; Carbohydrates: 30.9 g; Fiber: 8.9 g; Sugar: 6.2 g; Protein: 26.6 g

## Cinnamon Rice Meatballs

1 small onion
1 pound lean ground beef
½ cup uncooked rice
½ cup + ½ cup water
¼ teaspoon celery salt
¼ teaspoon salt
¼ teaspoon pepper
¼ teaspoon garlic powder
¾ teaspoon dried mint flakes
1 tablespoon dried parsley flakes
½ teaspoon cinnamon
1 (15-ounce) can tomato sauce

1. Preheat oven to 350°F. Spray an 8″ × 12″ baking pan with nonstick spray.
2. Peel off the outer skin of the onion, and throw it away. Chop the onion into very small pieces.
3. In a medium bowl, mix the onion, ground beef, rice, ½ cup of water, celery salt, salt, pepper, garlic powder, mint, and parsley. (The easiest way to mix this is with your hands.)
4. With your hands, shape the meat mixture into balls about the size of Ping-Pong balls.
5. Place the meatballs in the baking pan.
6. In a small bowl, stir together the cinnamon, ½ cup of water, and the tomato sauce. Spoon this sauce over the meatballs.
7. Cover the baking pan with foil. Bake for 45 minutes. Uncover the pan and bake 15 minutes longer.

*Makes 4 (5-meatball) servings*

One serving—Calories: 259; Total fat: 5.8 g; Saturated fat: 2.5 g; Cholesterol: 218 mg; Sodium: 397 mg; Carbohydrates: 24.1 g; Fiber: 1.9 g; Sugar: 3.4 g; Protein: 26.3 g

## All-in-One Dinner

1 (10-ounce) box frozen chopped spinach, thawed

½ green pepper, chopped into small pieces

1 onion, chopped into small pieces

1 pound lean ground beef

1 (15-ounce) can diced tomatoes, undrained

2 cans (8 ounces each) tomato sauce

1 cup uncooked rice

½ cup grated Monterey Jack cheese (Vegan Gourmet Monterey Jack Cheese Alternative is dairy-free)

¾ teaspoon chili powder

½ teaspoon salt

½ teaspoon black pepper

1¼ cups water

1. Preheat oven to 400°F. Spray a 2-quart casserole with nonstick spray.
2. Squeeze the spinach dry. Place it in a large bowl. Add the green pepper and onion.
3. With your hands, crumble the ground beef into the bowl.
4. Add the tomatoes, tomato sauce, rice, cheese, chili powder, salt, black pepper, and water. Stir well to blend, breaking up meat and spinach with the edge of a spoon.
5. Spoon the mixture into the casserole. Pack it down lightly, and smooth the surface.
6. Cover the casserole with a lid or foil. Bake for 1¼ hours.

*Makes 6 (1½-cup) servings*

One serving—Calories: 314; Total fat: 7.4 g; Saturated fat: 3.6 g; Cholesterol: 248 mg; Sodium: 663 mg; Carbohydrates: 38.9 g; Fiber: 5 g; Sugar: 4.9 g; Protein: 24.4 g

## Beefy Bean and Tater Casserole

1 pound lean ground beef

½ cup chopped onion

1 (14½-ounce) can French-style green beans, drained

1 (15-ounce) can diced tomatoes

¾ teaspoon salt

¼ teaspoon pepper

1 teaspoon chili powder

2 teaspoons sugar

2 teaspoons cornstarch

1½ tablespoons gluten-free Worcestershire sauce (Lea & Perrins Worcestershire Sauce is gluten- and dairy-free in the United States; the Canadian version has malt added and is not gluten-free)

1 (32-ounce) bag frozen Tater Tot potatoes (Ore-Ida Tater Tots are gluten- and dairy-free)

1 Preheat oven to 350°F. Spray a 9″ × 13″ baking dish with non-stick spray.

2 Place the beef and onion in a large microwave-safe bowl; cover the bowl with wax paper, and microwave for 1 minute. Remove bowl and break up meat with a fork. Continue to microwave for 5 minutes or until the onion is softened and the meat is browned, removing the dish once every minute to continue breaking up the meat. Throw away the wax paper and drain off any fat in the bowl.

3 Stir in the remaining ingredients except the potatoes. Spoon the mixture into the baking dish, and then top with the Tater Tots.

4 Bake for 30 minutes.

*Makes 4 (1-cup) servings*

One serving—Calories: 577; Total fat: 23.6 g; Saturated fat: 6.4 g; Cholesterol: 68 mg; Sodium: 1,241 mg; Carbohydrates: 61.8 g; Fiber: 6.9 g; Sugar: 4.8 g; Protein: 28.5 g

## Barbeque Roast

2 tablespoons cider vinegar

2 tablespoons brown sugar

1 teaspoon cornstarch

1¼ cups ketchup (Del Monte ketchup is gluten- and dairy-free)

2 teaspoons chili powder

¼ teaspoon salt

¼ teaspoon black pepper

1 tablespoon dried onion flakes

¼ cup chopped green pepper

1 cup water

1 (2-pound) boneless chuck roast

1 Preheat oven to 350°F.

2 In a medium bowl, stir together the vinegar, brown sugar, and cornstarch. Add the ketchup, chili powder, salt, black pepper,

onion flakes, and green pepper. Stir in the water. Pour half of this mixture over the bottom of a roasting pan.

③ Cut the roast into six serving pieces, then place in the roasting pan over the sauce. Pour the remaining sauce over the top of the roast.

④ Cover the pan with foil and bake for 3 hours or until the meat flakes easily with a fork, adding more water as needed.

*Makes 6 servings*

One serving—Calories: 444; Total fat: 27.5 g; Saturated fat: 11 g; Cholesterol: 100 mg; Sodium: 755 mg; Carbohydrates: 18.7 g; Fiber: 0.6 g; Sugar: 16.4 g; Protein: 30.2 g

# No-Fuss Beef Roast

1 cup medium-hot salsa

¼ teaspoon salt

¼ teaspoon black pepper

¼ teaspoon garlic powder

1 tablespoon dried parsley flakes

1 tablespoon oregano

1 teaspoon gluten-free beef bouillon granules (Herb-Ox granules are gluten- and dairy-free)

½ cup sliced carrot

1 medium onion, sliced

1 rib celery, sliced

¼ green pepper, sliced thin

2 teaspoons cornstarch

¾ cup water

2 pounds chuck beef roast

① Preheat oven to 350°F.

② Cut a piece of heavy-duty foil that is a little more than double the length of a 9-inch square baking pan. Place the foil inside the pan, letting the ends hang out.

③ In a bowl, stir together the salsa, salt, black pepper, garlic powder, parsley, oregano, bouillon granules, carrot, onion, celery, green pepper, and cornstarch. Stir in the water.

④ Spoon one-quarter of the sauce into the foil-lined pan. Place the beef roast in the pan on top of the sauce. Carefully pour the remaining sauce on the roast.

⑤ Bring foil overhangs up to the center, and fold them together securely. Fold the sides of the foil securely so the roast is totally sealed.

⑥ Roast for 3 hours or until the meat is very tender. Be careful opening up the foil because hot steam will escape.

*Makes 6 servings*

One serving—Calories: 414; Total fat: 28.3 g; Saturated fat: 11.4 g; Cholesterol: 103 mg; Sodium: 684 mg; Carbohydrates: 8.5 g; Fiber: 2.6 g; Sugar: 4.4 g; Protein: 29.7 g

## Corned Beef and Cabbage

6 large red-skinned potatoes, each cut into 4 wedges

1 (2-pound) lean corned beef brisket

8 whole black peppercorns

2 bay leaves

1 small head of cabbage

6 teaspoons butter

① Place the potatoes on the bottom of a large slow cooker. Carefully cut most of the visible fat from the corned beef. (A child may need an adult to help with this.) If the roast is too large to fit in the slow cooker, cut it into two pieces. Put the corned beef on top of the potatoes. Sprinkle the peppercorns and bay leaves on top.

② Cut the cabbage into six wedges. Remove the hard center core from each wedge. Put the cabbage wedges on top of the meat. Add enough water to just barely cover the cabbage. Cook on low heat for 8 hours.

③ With a slotted spoon, remove the cabbage to six serving dishes. Remove the meat; slice it against the grain, then set it on the six serving dishes. Remove the potatoes with a slotted spoon and divide them among the six serving dishes. Place ½ teaspoon butter on each stack of potatoes and ½ teaspoon butter on each cabbage wedge. Serve with mustard, if desired.

**Note:** The corned beef shrinks to about half its original size while cooking.

*Makes 6 servings (¼ pound cooked brisket plus 1 potato and ⅙ head of cabbage)*

One serving—Calories: 567; Total fat: 32.2 g; Saturated fat: 14.1 g; Cholesterol: 135 mg; Sodium: 1,321 mg; Carbohydrates: 46 g; Fiber: 7.6 g; Sugar: 8 g; Protein: 26.2 g

## Fun Fajitas

¾ cup mild or medium salsa

¼ teaspoon cumin

¼ teaspoon salt

¼ teaspoon black pepper

¼ teaspoon garlic powder

1 medium onion, sliced thin

½ green pepper, sliced thin

1 tablespoon + 1 tablespoon olive oil

6 ounces chicken tenders

4 (8-inch) gluten-free flour tortillas (Don Pancho flour tortillas are gluten- and dairy-free)

¾ cup cheddar cheese (Vegan Gourmet Cheddar Cheese Alternative is dairy-free)

① In a medium bowl, stir together the salsa, cumin, salt, black pepper, and garlic powder; set aside.

② In a large nonstick skillet, sauté onion and green pepper in 1 tablespoon olive oil, over medium-high heat, about 2 minutes or just until tender crisp; remove the onion and green pepper to a plate.

3 Put the chicken strips into the same skillet, adding the remaining 1 tablespoon olive oil, and sauté over medium-high heat, stirring frequently, until the chicken is just cooked through, about 5 minutes.

4 Wrap the tortillas in a damp paper towel and microwave for 15 seconds to soften them.

5 Lay one tortilla on each of four plates. Lay the chicken strips down the center of each tortilla, dividing them evenly. Top each tortilla with one-fourth of the onions and green peppers. Spoon one-fourth of the salsa mixture over each, then top each with one-fourth of the cheese. Fold in the sides to hold in the filling, and then roll up the tortilla.

*Makes 4 (1-tortilla) servings*

One serving—Calories: 438; Total fat: 23.6 g; Saturated fat: 7.2 g; Cholesterol: 40 mg; Sodium: 1,064 mg; Carbohydrates: 38.5 g; Fiber: 2.8 g; Sugar: 4.8 g; Protein: 16.5 g

## Buffalo Wings

10 buffalo wings (5 whole chicken wings cut at the joint; discard the wing tips)

1 cup water

½ cup balsamic vinegar

⅓ cup gluten-free soy sauce (San-J Premium Tamari Soy Sauce is gluten- and dairy-free)

2½ tablespoons sugar

1 clove garlic, peeled and sliced lengthwise into 4 pieces

1 small hot chili pepper, cut in half, seeds removed

1 Place all of the ingredients in a medium-size saucepan.

2 Over high heat, bring the mixture to a boil. Then lower the heat to medium and simmer for about 25 minutes or until the wings are tender.

3 Turn the heat to high and cook for 5 more minutes to reduce the sauce so it thickens. Remove the garlic and hot pepper before serving.

*Makes 2 (5-piece) servings*

One serving—Calories: 265; Total fat: 8.2 g; Saturated fat: 2.3 g; Cholesterol: 33 mg; Sodium: 1,708 mg; Carbohydrates: 30.7 g; Fiber: 0.6 g; Sugar: 27 g; Protein: 14.9 g

## 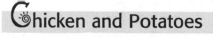hicken and Potatoes

4 bone-in chicken breasts

5 cloves garlic

4 large red-skinned potatoes

1 lemon

⅓ cup olive oil

1 (14-ounce) can gluten-free chicken broth (Swanson Chicken Broth is gluten- and dairy-free)

½ teaspoon salt

¼ teaspoon pepper

¼ teaspoon dried mint flakes

1½ teaspoons dried oregano

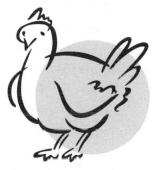

1 Preheat oven to 350°F.

2 Place the chicken in an 8″ × 12″ baking dish.

3 Peel the skin off the garlic cloves. Cut the cloves in half lengthwise. Scatter the cut cloves around the chicken.

4 Cut the potatoes in half lengthwise. Cut each half lengthwise into four pieces. Place the potatoes around the chicken.

5 Cut the lemon in half. With a fork, squeeze the juice from the lemon into a small bowl. Remove any seeds from the bowl. Sprinkle the lemon juice over the chicken and potatoes.

6 Drizzle the olive oil over the potatoes and chicken.

7 Pour the broth over the chicken.

8 Sprinkle the potatoes and chicken with the salt, pepper, mint flakes, and oregano.

9 Bake uncovered for 1 hour or until the chicken and potatoes are very tender. (If most of the pan juices evaporate, add ¾ cup very hot water to the pan halfway through cooking.)

*Makes 4 servings*

One serving—Calories: 413; Total fat: 27.7 g; Saturated fat: 5.5 g; Cholesterol: 85 mg; Sodium: 376 mg; Carbohydrates: 11.7 g; Fiber: 1.6 g; Sugar: 1 g; Protein: 28.7 g

## Finger-Lickin' Great Chicken Nuggets

¼ cup honey

2 tablespoons water

2 tablespoons olive oil

1 cup crushed gluten-free puffed rice cereal (Morning Puffs Honey
     & Maple Rice Puffs are gluten- and dairy-free)

¼ teaspoon salt

¼ teaspoon pepper

½ teaspoon paprika

1 pound boneless, skinless chicken tenders

1 In a medium bowl, stir together the honey, water, and oil.

2 Put the crushed cereal, salt, pepper, and paprika into a quart-size self-seal bag.

3 Stir the chicken tenders into the honey mixture to evenly coat all of the pieces.

4 Next put the chicken tenders into the self-seal bag, seal the bag, then shake the bag well to coat all of the pieces with the cereal crumbs.

5 Spray a baking sheet with nonstick spray. Place the chicken tenders onto the baking sheet, cover with foil, and refrigerate the baking sheet for 2 or more hours to set the crumb mixture.

6 Preheat the oven to 425°F.

7. Bake the chicken pieces for 10 minutes or until they are cooked through. Do not overcook or the chicken may become tough. There is no need to turn the pieces during baking.

**Note:** To crush the cereal easily, put it in a self-seal plastic bag, then use a rolling pin to crush the rice puffs.

*Makes 4 (¼-pound) servings*

One serving—Calories: 217; Total fat: 7.6 g; Saturated fat: 1.1 g; Cholesterol: 34 mg; Sodium: 248 mg; Carbohydrates: 23.7 g; Fiber: 0.2 g; Sugar: 18.1 g; Protein: 14.2 g

## Stuffed Chicken Roll

4 boneless, skinless chicken breasts (5 ounces each)

8 thin slices green pepper

2 thin green onions sliced in half crosswise, then sliced into thin strips lengthwise

8 (3-ounce) slices Monterey Jack cheese (Vegan Gourmet Monterey Jack Cheese Alternative is dairy-free)

1 (4-ounce) can sliced mushrooms, drained

1 tablespoon olive oil

2½ tablespoons cornstarch

¾ cup milk (use casein-free soy or rice milk for dairy-free diets)

1½ cups gluten-free chicken broth (Swanson Chicken Broth is gluten- and dairy-free)

1 envelope gluten-free dry onion soup mix (Lipton Onion Soup Mix is gluten- and dairy-free)

1 tablespoon dried parsley flakes

½ teaspoon salt

½ teaspoon black pepper

1 teaspoon paprika

1. Preheat oven to 350°F. Spray a 9-inch square pan with nonstick spray.

2. On a cutting board, using a meat mallet, pound the chicken breasts until they are fairly thin.

③ Lay two slices of green pepper, two slices of onion, and two slices of cheese at one end of each of the chicken breasts. Fold the end of the breast in, then roll up the breast, sealing in the green pepper, onion, and cheese; secure with toothpicks. Set the rolled breasts in the baking pan.

④ In a medium-size saucepan, brown the mushrooms in the oil over medium-high heat, stirring frequently. Spoon the browned mushrooms over the chicken.

⑤ In a medium-size bowl, stir together the cornstarch and ¼ cup milk until mixture is smooth. Stir in the remaining milk. Pour this mixture into the saucepan used to brown the mushrooms, scraping up any browned bits from the bottom of the pan. Stir in the broth, soup mix, parsley flakes, salt, pepper, and paprika, and cook over medium heat, stirring constantly, until mixture begins to thicken. Pour this sauce over the chicken breasts and mushrooms.

⑥ Bake for 30 minutes or until the chicken is cooked through.

**Note:** Adults may want to use slices of hot banana peppers in place of the green pepper and stir ½ cup sherry into the sauce after the sauce has thickened.

*Makes 4 servings*

One serving—Calories: 487; Total fat: 25.6 g; Saturated fat: 9.4 g; Cholesterol: 118 mg; Sodium: 1,745 mg; Carbohydrates: 22.7 g; Fiber: 4.6 g; Sugar: 7.6 g; Protein: 41.7 g

## Chicken Kabobs

In place of the chicken, you can use lean pork, ham cubes, or raw shrimp.

1 pound boneless, skinless chicken breasts

¼ cup Italian dressing

2 tablespoons gluten-free soy sauce (San-J Premium Tamari Soy Sauce is gluten- and dairy-free)

⅛ teaspoon black pepper

½ green pepper

1 medium onion

8 pineapple chunks

1. If you are using wooden skewers, soak them in water for 30 minutes. (This keeps them from burning on the grill.)

2. Wash the chicken. Cut it into ¾-inch squares. Put the chicken in a quart-size, reclosable plastic bag.

3. Add the dressing, soy sauce, and black pepper to the bag. Seal the bag. Gently push the chicken pieces around so the marinade distributes evenly. Refrigerate chicken for at least 1 hour.

4. Remove the white membrane and seeds from inside the green pepper and discard. Cut the pepper into four pieces. Peel the onion, then cut it into four wedges.

5. Thread the skewers with chicken, green pepper, pineapple, and onion, dividing the ingredients evenly. Throw away any leftover marinade.

6. An adult should preheat the grill, and then spray it with a nonstick spray. Grill the kabobs for about 10 minutes, turning frequently. Use tongs to turn the chicken. (Instead of grilling, kabobs may be broiled.)

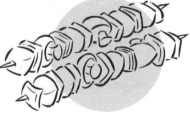

*Makes 4 kabobs*

One kabob—Calories: 210; Total fat: 5.7 g; Saturated fat: 1.1 g; Cholesterol: 68 mg; Sodium: 824 mg; Carbohydrates: 10.1 g; Fiber: 1.1 g; Sugar: 6.6 g; Protein: 28.8 g

## Baked Chicken Stew

4 whole chicken legs (or 4 bone-in chicken breasts)

4 large red-skinned potatoes, cut into 1-inch cubes

1 medium onion, cut into thin wedges

1 cup frozen cut green beans

1 cup frozen peas

20 baby carrots

3 cups spaghetti sauce (Emeril's Home Style Marinara Sauce is
gluten- and dairy-free)

1 cup water

1 tablespoon olive oil

1 teaspoon minced garlic

½ teaspoon cinnamon

½ teaspoon salt

½ teaspoon pepper

1 teaspoon Italian seasoning

1. Preheat oven to 375°F. Spray a 9″ × 13″ baking pan with non-stick spray.

2. Wash the chicken pieces, removing all visible fat. Place the chicken pieces in the baking pan.

3. Add the potatoes, onion, green beans, peas, and carrots around the chicken pieces.

4. In a medium bowl, stir together the spaghetti sauce, water, oil, garlic, cinnamon, salt, pepper, and Italian seasoning. Pour this mixture over the chicken and vegetables.

5. Bake for 2 hours or until the chicken is fork-tender, adding more water if needed.

*Makes 4 servings*

One serving—Calories: 569; Total fat: 18.8 g; Saturated fat: 4.6 g; Cholesterol: 67 mg; Sodium: 1,094 mg; Carbohydrates: 70.8 g; Fiber: 11.3 g; Sugar: 23.1 g; Protein: 28.3 g

## Easy Baked Chicken

¼ cup gluten-free flour mixture (See the
Gluten-Free Flour Mixtures on
page 16)

¼ teaspoon salt

¼ teaspoon pepper

4 whole chicken legs

4 tablespoons butter, melted (use dairy-free margarine for dairy-free diets)

1 cup half-and-half (use casein-free soy or rice milk for dairy-free diets)

1. Preheat oven to 375°F. Spray an 8½″ × 11″ baking pan with nonstick spray.
2. In a large self-seal bag, mix together the flour mixture, salt, and pepper.
3. Add the chicken to the bag. Seal the bag and shake it well to cover the pieces evenly with flour. Remove the chicken and place the pieces in the baking dish.
4. Pour the melted butter (or margarine) over the chicken pieces.
5. Pour the half-and-half over the chicken pieces.
6. Bake for ½ hour, then turn the chicken pieces. Bake for another ½ hour or until the chicken is fork-tender.

**Note:** You can make an alternative version for adults: pour ½ cup sherry over the chicken before adding the half-and-half.

*Makes 4 servings*

One serving  Calories: 370; Total fat. 27.8 g; Saturated fat: 14.2 g; Cholesterol: 116 mg; Sodium: 312 mg; Carbohydrates: 9.5 g; Fiber: 0.4 g; Sugar: 0.1 g; Protein: 20.1 g

## Baked Ham

1 tablespoon brown sugar

2 tablespoons maple syrup

2 tablespoons brown mustard

2 boneless ham slices (about 1 pound total)

¼ cup water

1. Preheat oven to 325°F. Spray a shallow baking dish with nonstick spray.
2. In a small bowl, stir together the brown sugar, maple syrup, and brown mustard.

3 Lay the ham slices in the baking dish, then spread each slice with the brown sugar mixture.

4 Pour the water around the sides of the ham slices (not over the top). Cover the pan with foil and bake for 25 minutes.

*Makes 2 servings*

One serving—Calories: 285; Total fat: 8 g; Saturated fat: 2.4 g; Cholesterol: 93 mg; Sodium: 1,590 mg; Carbohydrates: 21.7 g; Fiber: 0.5 g; Sugar: 20.3 g; Protein: 32.8 g

# Stuffed Ham Slices

3 slices gluten-free bread, toasted and cut into ¼-inch cubes
    (Ener-G Foods Four Flour Loaf is gluten- and dairy-free)
½ teaspoon cinnamon
2 tablespoons honey
2 tablespoons brown sugar
½ can (½ of a 21-ounce can) apple pie filling (Comstock apple pie
    filling is gluten- and dairy-free)
2 tablespoons raisins
4 slices boneless ham (about 2 pounds total)

1 Preheat oven to 325 degrees. Spray a 9″ × 13″ baking pan with nonstick spray.

2 In a bowl, stir together the bread cubes, cinnamon, honey, brown sugar, pie filling, and raisins.

3 Place two ham slices in the baking pan. Spread the stuffing mix on top of the slices, dividing evenly. Top with the remaining two ham slices.

4 Cover the pan with foil and bake for 35 minutes. To serve, cut each stuffed ham in half.

*Makes 4 servings*

One serving—Calories: 393; Total fat: 8.4 g; Saturated fat: 2.5 g; Cholesterol: 93 mg; Sodium: 1,543 mg; Carbohydrates: 48.1 g; Fiber: 2.1 g; Sugar: 30.7 g; Protein: 34.2 g

# Pork Chops and Beans

1 (28-ounce) can gluten-free baked beans
    (Bush's Original Baked Beans are
    gluten- and dairy-free)
2 tablespoons brown sugar
3 tablespoons molasses
1 tablespoon yellow mustard
4 loin pork chops, 5 ounces each
1 onion, sliced thin
¼ teaspoon salt
¼ teaspoon pepper

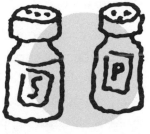

1. Preheat oven to 350°F. Spray an 8″ × 11″ baking pan with nonstick spray.
2. Spoon the beans into the baking pan. Stir in the brown sugar, molasses, and mustard.
3. Place the pork chops on top of the beans, then lay the onion slices on top of the meat. Sprinkle salt and pepper on top of the onions.
4. Cover the pan with foil and bake for 1 hour 20 minutes.
5. Remove pan from oven and turn on the broiler. Broil the casserole for 8 minutes or until the onions are beginning to brown.

*Makes 4 (1 chop + 7 ounces beans) servings*

One serving—Calories: 390; Total fat: 11.9 g; Saturated fat: 4 g; Cholesterol: 87 mg; Sodium: 721 mg; Carbohydrates: 40.9 g; Fiber: 5.8 g; Sugar: 19.6 g; Protein: 32.7 g

# Pork Chops with Apples

2 tablespoons + 2 tablespoons gluten-free brown mustard
    (French's Spicy Brown Mustard is gluten- and dairy-free)
2 pork chops, 5 ounces each

¼ teaspoon salt
¼ teaspoon pepper
1 medium onion, sliced thin
1 apple, peeled and cored
⅓ cup honey

1. Preheat oven to 350°F. Spray a shallow 1-quart baking dish with nonstick spray.
2. With a blunt knife, spread 1 tablespoon mustard on one side of each of the pork chops. Sprinkle the coated sides with half of the salt and pepper. Place the chops, mustard-side down, into the baking dish.
3. Spread the remaining 2 tablespoons mustard on top of the chops; sprinkle with the remaining salt and pepper.
4. Lay the sliced onion on top of the pork chops.
5. Slice the apple in half, and then cut each half into thin slices. Lay the apple slices on top of the onions.
6. Drizzle the honey over the tops of the apples.
7. Bake uncovered for 1 hour.

*Makes 2 (1-chop) servings*

One serving—Calories: 505; Total fat: 14.7 g; Saturated fat: 4.7 g; Cholesterol: 103 mg; Sodium: 756 mg; Carbohydrates: 76.7 g; Fiber: 3.1 g; Sugar: 56.7 g; Protein: 33.4 g

## Baked Cornmeal Hot Dogs

1 egg
½ cup milk (use casein-free soy or rice milk for dairy-free diets)
1 teaspoon olive oil
½ teaspoon prepared mustard (Gulden's Spicy Brown Mustard is gluten- and dairy-free)
2 tablespoons brown sugar
2 teaspoons baking powder
1 teaspoon baking soda
½ teaspoon dry mustard

¼ teaspoon salt

⅔ cup fine cornmeal

½ cup gluten-free flour mixture (See the Gluten-Free Flour Mixtures on page 16)

8 gluten-free hot dogs (Shelton's hot dogs are gluten- and dairy-free)

1. Preheat oven to 400°F. Spray a baking sheet with nonstick spray.

2. In a medium mixing bowl, whisk the egg until frothy. Add the milk, oil, and prepared mustard; whisk till blended.

3. Whisk in the brown sugar, baking powder, baking soda, dry mustard, and salt.

4. Using a rubber spatula, blend in the cornmeal and flour mixture. The batter will be thick.

5. Insert a small skewer lengthwise into each of the hot dogs, pushing the skewer in as far as possible while leaving 2½ inches of the skewer exposed for picking up the hot dogs. Dip each hot dog into the batter. With wet fingers, form the batter around each hot dog until most of the hot dog is covered. Place coated hot dogs on the baking sheet.

6. Bake for 15 minutes or until puffed and golden.

**Note:** Use a finely ground cornmeal for this recipe for good results.

*Makes 8 corn dogs*

One corn dog—Calories: 152; Total fat: 2.3 g; Saturated fat: 0.7 g; Cholesterol: 42 mg; Sodium: 828 mg; Carbohydrates: 23.7 g; Fiber: 0.9 g; Sugar: 5.5 g; Protein: 8.8 g

# Hot Dog Burrito

1 egg

1 tablespoon milk (use casein-free soy or rice milk for dairy-free diets)

Dash pepper

1 gluten-free hot dog (Hebrew National hot dogs are gluten- and casein-free)

1 teaspoon butter (use dairy-free margarine for dairy-free diets)

1 slice cheddar cheese (Vegan Gourmet Cheddar Cheese Alternative is dairy-free)

1 gluten-free corn tortilla (Mission corn tortillas are gluten- and dairy-free)

1 teaspoon ketchup (Del Monte and Heinz ketchups are gluten- and dairy-free)

1. In a bowl, whisk together the egg, milk, and pepper.
2. Thinly slice the hot dog.
3. Melt the butter or margarine in a small skillet.
4. Add the hot dog slices to the skillet. Cook, stirring often, for 1 minute.
5. Add the egg mixture to the pan. Cook, stirring constantly, until the egg is cooked.
6. Place the cheese on top of the tortilla.
7. Spread the ketchup on top of the cheese. Spoon on the egg and hot dog mixture.
8. Roll your "sandwich" up like a burrito.

*Makes 1 burrito*

One burrito—Calories: 424; Total fat: 30.3 g; Saturated fat: 14.9 g; Cholesterol: 276 mg; Sodium: 928 mg; Carbohydrates: 15.7 g; Fiber: 1.4 g; Sugar: 2.5 g; Protein: 22.2 g

# 6

# Side Dishes

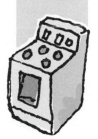

## Hot Side Dishes

### Mini Carrot Fries

2 cups mini carrots
1¼ teaspoons brown sugar
1½ tablespoons olive oil
½ teaspoon salt
⅛ teaspoon pepper
¼ teaspoon cinnamon

1 Preheat oven to 425°F. Lightly spray a baking sheet with non-stick spray.

2 Cut each carrot lengthwise in half, and then cut each half in half again to get four lengthwise pieces from each carrot. Place the carrot slices into a medium bowl.

3 Add the brown sugar, oil, salt, pepper, and cinnamon to the bowl and stir until the carrots are evenly coated.

4 Spoon the carrots onto the baking pan, spreading them out in a single layer so they don't overlap.

5 Bake for 15 to 20 minutes or until the carrots are tender.

*Makes 4 (½-cup) servings*

One serving—Calories: 76; Total fat: 5.2 g; Saturated fat: 0.7 g; Cholesterol: 0 mg; Sodium: 333 mg; Carbohydrates: 7.4 g; Fiber: 1.8 g; Sugar: 4.3 g; Protein: 0.6 g

## Mexican Rice

1 small onion

1 cup uncooked long-grain rice

2 tablespoons olive oil

2 tablespoons canned, chopped green chilies

1 cup very hot water

1 teaspoon gluten-free chicken bouillon granules (Herb-Ox makes
   gluten-free, dairy-free bouillon granules)

1 cup salsa

1 Peel and chop the onion.

2 Cook the onion and rice in the oil in a medium saucepan over medium heat, stirring frequently, until the rice is golden.

3 Add the chilies, hot water, bouillon granules, and salsa, stirring until blended. Cover the pan, and lower the heat. Let the rice steam for 15 to 20 minutes until all the liquid is absorbed.

*Makes 4 (¾-cup) servings*

One serving—Calories: 256; Total fat: 7.1 g; Saturated fat: 1 g; Cholesterol: 0 mg; Sodium: 581 mg; Carbohydrates: 43.5 g; Fiber: 3.2 g; Sugar: 5.3 g; Protein: 3.6 g

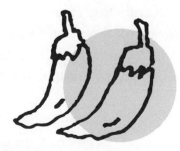

# Spinach and Rice

2 boxes (10 ounces each) frozen chopped spinach, thawed

¾ cup uncooked rice

½ cup tomato sauce

1¾ cups water

3 tablespoons olive oil

1 tablespoon dill weed

¼ teaspoon salt

¼ teaspoon pepper

1 tablespoon dried minced onion

1. Preheat oven to 350°F. Spray an 8-inch square pan with non-stick spray.
2. Squeeze the spinach dry. Put it in a medium bowl.
3. Add the rice to the bowl, and stir with a fork, breaking up the spinach.
4. Put the tomato sauce, water, olive oil, dill, salt, pepper, and minced onion in a small saucepan. Put the pan on the stove, and bring it to a boil over high heat.
5. Remove the pan and pour the sauce over the spinach and rice. Stir to blend well.
6. Spoon the spinach mixture into the baking pan. Bake for 30 minutes or until the rice is tender and most of the liquid has been absorbed.

**Note:** All plain rice is gluten-free, but some prepackaged flavored rice (such as Rice-a-Roni) is not. Almost any plain rice can be used in this recipe (white, brown, basmati, etc.).

*Makes 6 (2½" × 4") servings*

One serving—Calories: 181; Total fat: 11.3 g; Saturated fat: 1.4 g; Cholesterol: 0 mg; Sodium: 276 mg; Carbohydrates: 24.6 g; Fiber: 3.5 g; Sugar: 1.8 g; Protein: 5.5 g

## Polka-Dot Rice

2¼ cups water

2 gluten-free beef bouillon cubes (Herb-Ox bouillon cubes are
    gluten- and dairy-free)

⅛ teaspoon pepper

1 tablespoon dried parsley flakes

⅓ cup frozen peas

1 cup uncooked rice

1. Put the water, bouillon cubes, pepper, and parsley in a medium saucepan. Bring to a boil on the stove.
2. When the water is boiling, stir in the peas and rice. Lower heat to simmer, and cover the pan with a lid. Simmer about 15 minutes or until all the water is absorbed.

*Makes 4 (½-cup) servings*

One serving—Calories: 183; Total fat: 0.5 g; Saturated fat: 0.2 g; Cholesterol: 0 mg; Sodium: 372 mg; Carbohydrates: 39.2 g; Fiber: 1.2 g; Sugar: 0.9 g; Protein: 4.3 g

## Spaghetti Squash

1 small spaghetti squash (about 1 pound)

¼ cup olive oil

3 tablespoons grated Parmesan cheese (Eat in the Raw Parma!
    Vegan Parmesan is gluten- and dairy-free)

½ cup shredded mozzarella cheese (Vegan Gourmet Mozzarella
    Cheese Alternative is gluten- and dairy-free)

12 cherry tomatoes, quartered

¼ teaspoon salt

⅛ teaspoon pepper

⅛ teaspoon oregano

1 tablespoon dried parsley

1. Cut off the flower end of the squash, then cut the squash in half lengthwise. (This is not easy to do. Children should not do this step themselves.)

2. Remove and throw away the seeds and tough fiber in the center of each half. Set the squash halves, cut side up, on a large microwave-safe dish, then cover with wax paper.

3. Microwave the squash on high for 15 minutes. Remove from the microwave (it will be very hot, so use pot holders) and let it stand for 5 minutes.

4. Using a fork, scrape the insides of the squash to form strands. Place the strands into a medium bowl. Discard all but one of the squash shells.

5. Gently toss the oil, cheeses, tomatoes, salt, pepper, oregano, and parsley into the squash strands, and then spoon this mixture into the remaining squash shell.

6. Place the filled shell on a microwave-safe dish and microwave on high for 4 minutes or until the filling is heated through.

*Makes 4 (1-cup) servings*

One serving—Calories: 230; Total fat: 17.9 g; Saturated fat: 4.4 g; Cholesterol: 11 mg; Sodium: 309 mg; Carbohydrates: 13 g; Fiber: 2.9 g; Sugar: 5.4 g; Protein: 6.7 g

## Breaded Veggies

1 cup broccoli florets, cut into bite-size pieces

1 cup whole, fresh button mushrooms

1 cup cauliflower florets, cut into bite-size pieces

3 cups gluten-free cornflake crumbs (Nature's Path cornflakes are gluten- and dairy-free)

¼ teaspoon salt

Dash pepper

½ teaspoon Italian seasoning

¼ teaspoon garlic powder

¼ teaspoon paprika

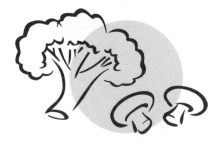

3 tablespoons grated Parmesan cheese (Eat in the Raw Parma!
    Vegan Parmesan is gluten- and dairy-free)

3 tablespoons Italian dressing

½ cup mayonnaise

1. Preheat oven to 425°F. Spray a baking sheet with nonstick spray.
2. Wash the broccoli, mushrooms, and cauliflower florets. Pat them dry with a paper towel.
3. Put the cereal crumbs in a quart-size, self-seal plastic bag. Add the salt, pepper, Italian seasoning, garlic powder, paprika, and cheese to the cereal bag. Seal the bag, and shake well to mix ingredients. (Before sealing bags used to mix ingredients, try to push out as much air as possible. This will make it easier to blend the ingredients inside the bag.)
4. In another quart-size, self-seal plastic bag, place the Italian dressing and mayonnaise. Seal the bag well. Press the contents to blend. Add the vegetable pieces. Reseal the bag, then shake the bag to evenly coat the vegetables.
5. Transfer the vegetables to the cereal bag. Seal the bag, and then shake it well to evenly coat the vegetables with the cereal crumb mixture.
6. Place the veggies on the baking sheet. Bake for 10 minutes or until lightly browned.

*Makes 4 (¾-cup) servings*

One serving—Calories: 266; Total fat: 14.6 g; Saturated fat: 2.7 g; Cholesterol: 11 mg; Sodium: 812 mg; Carbohydrates: 38.4 g; Fiber: 2.5 g; Sugar: 5.8 g; Protein: 3.7 g

## Corn Casserole

½ cup milk (use casein-free soy or rice milk for dairy-free diets)

2 teaspoons cornstarch

1 egg

½ teaspoon sugar

¼ teaspoon salt

1 tablespoon butter, melted (use dairy-free margarine for dairy-free diets)

1 (15¼-ounce) can corn, drained

¼ cup crushed corn chips (Tostitos are gluten-free and dairy-free)

1. Preheat oven to 350°F. Spray a 1-quart baking dish with non-stick spray.
2. In a medium bowl, whisk together the milk and cornstarch. Add the egg and whisk until light and frothy.
3. Whisk in the sugar, salt, and melted butter.
4. With a spoon, stir in the corn.
5. Spoon the corn mixture into the baking dish.
6. Sprinkle the crushed corn chips on top of the casserole.
7. Bake 30 minutes or until the mixture is set and just beginning to brown around the edges.

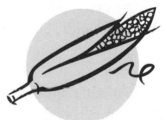

*Makes 4 (¾-cup) servings*

One serving—Calories: 171; Total fat: 7.3 g; Saturated fat: 3.1 g; Cholesterol: 64 mg; Sodium: 438 mg; Carbohydrates: 24.4 g; Fiber: 1.8 g; Sugar: 4.6 g; Protein: 5.1 g

## Potato and Broccoli Casserole

1 (10-ounce) box frozen chopped broccoli

1 egg, slightly beaten

1¼ cups milk (use casein-free soy or rice milk for dairy-free diets)

¾ cup water

¼ cup olive oil

¼ teaspoon garlic powder

2 teaspoons dried onion flakes

¼ teaspoon salt

¼ teaspoon pepper

1½ cups instant mashed potato flakes (Bob's Red Mill offers gluten-free, dairy-free instant mashed potatoes)

⅔ cup cheddar cheese (Vegan Gourmet Cheddar Cheese Alternative is gluten- and dairy-free)

⅛ teaspoon paprika

1 Preheat oven to 325°F. Spray an 8-inch pie pan with nonstick spray.

2 Place the opened box of broccoli on a microwave-safe plate and microwave on high for 6 minutes to defrost. Remove the hot dish with pot holders. Spoon the broccoli into a sieve, and then run cold water over the broccoli to cool it down. With your hands, picking up one handful of broccoli at a time, squeeze the water out of the broccoli, then place it in a large bowl.

3 Whisk the egg in a small bowl. Add the milk and whisk again to blend. Set the bowl aside.

4 Put the water, oil, garlic powder, onion flakes, salt, and pepper in a medium saucepan. Put the pan on the stove and cook on high. As soon as the water begins to boil, remove the pan and set it on a pot holder.

5 Using a fork, stir the potato flakes into the egg-milk mixture until well blended. Then stir in the broccoli and cheese.

6 Spoon the potato mixture into the pie plate. Sprinkle the top lightly with paprika.

7 Cover the pan with foil and bake for 20 minutes.

*Makes 6 (¾-cup) servings*

One serving—Calories: 165; Total fat: 18.3 g; Saturated fat: 6.9 g; Cholesterol: 61 mg; Sodium: 353 mg; Carbohydrates: 12.9 g; Fiber: 2.6 g; Sugar: 3.7 g; Protein: 8.3 g

# Hash Brown Casserole

1 (16-ounce) package gluten-free frozen hash brown potatoes,
   thawed

3 tablespoons canned, chopped green chilies

½ teaspoon salt

¼ teaspoon pepper

2 tablespoons dried parsley flakes

1 (14½-ounce) can stewed tomatoes, undrained

½ cup shredded cheddar cheese (Vegan Gourmet Cheddar Cheese
   Alternative is gluten- and dairy-free)

1. Spray a 2-quart, microwave-safe casserole with nonstick spray. Place the potatoes in the casserole.

2. Stir in the green chilies, salt, pepper, parsley, tomatoes (including the juice), and cheese. (If you want to make this casserole ahead, you can cover and refrigerate it for up to 8 hours, then bake just before dinnertime.)

3. Cover the casserole; microwave on high for 6 minutes.

4. Stir the ingredients. Return the casserole to the microwave for 8 more minutes on high.

**Note:** This casserole may be baked in the oven instead of the microwave. Before you prepare the casserole, preheat the oven to 400°F, then bake the casserole for 40 minutes.

*Makes 6 (¾-cup) servings*

One serving—Calories: 125; Total fat: 3.7 g; Saturated fat: 2.1 g; Cholesterol: 10 mg; Sodium: 437 mg; Carbohydrates: 18.2 g; Fiber: 1.9 g; Sugar: 2.6 g; Protein: 4.6 g

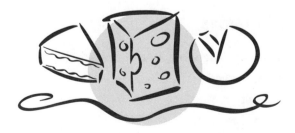

## Au Gratin Potatoes

1 (15-ounce) can whole potatoes, drained

⅓ cup milk (use soy or rice milk for dairy-free diets)

1 tablespoon olive oil

½ teaspoon brown mustard

¼ teaspoon salt

¼ teaspoon pepper

2 teaspoons cornstarch

1 cup shredded cheddar cheese (Vegan Gourmet Cheddar Cheese
   Alternative is gluten- and dairy-free)

1  Cut the potatoes into ½-inch cubes, then place them in a small saucepan.

2  In a small bowl, stir together the milk, oil, mustard, salt, pepper, cornstarch, and cheese. Spoon this mixture over the potatoes.

3  Cook over medium heat, stirring, until mixture is hot and sauce has been absorbed, about 10 minutes.

**Note:** There are two basic kinds of vegan cheddar cheese—one that melts easily and one that does not. In cold dishes, it doesn't make any difference which of these cheeses you use, but in recipes that are cooked, the melting kind of cheese is preferable. The package clearly states, "It melts!"

*Makes 4 (¾-cup) servings*

One serving—Calories: 206; Total fat: 13.5 g; Saturated fat: 6.8 g; Cholesterol: 32 mg; Sodium: 464 mg; Carbohydrates: 13 g; Fiber: 1.4 g; Sugar: 1.2 g; Protein: 8.6 g

## Creamy Potatoes

1 (16-ounce) bag gluten-free, frozen shredded hash brown
   potatoes, thawed

½ teaspoon salt

¼ teaspoon pepper

½ teaspoon garlic powder

1 tablespoon dried onion flakes

1 tablespoon dried parsley flakes

1 teaspoon brown mustard

1½ cups whole milk (use casein-free soy or
rice milk for dairy-free diets)

¾ cup shredded cheddar cheese (Vegan
Gourmet Cheddar Cheese Alternative is
gluten- and dairy-free)

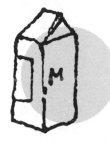

⅓ cup shredded Monterey Jack cheese
(Vegan Gourmet Monterey Jack Cheese
Alternative is gluten- and dairy-free)

1 cup gluten-free cornflake crumbs (Nature's Path cornflakes are
gluten- and dairy-free)

3 tablespoons olive oil

½ teaspoon paprika

1 Preheat oven to 350°F. Spray an 8″ × 11″ baking pan with
nonstick spray.

2 In a large bowl, stir together the potatoes, salt, pepper, garlic
powder, onion flakes, parsley, mustard, milk, and cheeses.

3 Spoon the potato mixture into the baking pan.

4 In a small bowl, stir together the cornflake crumbs, oil, and
paprika. Sprinkle the crumbs on top of the potatoes.

5 Bake for 55 minutes or until the potatoes are tender.

*Makes 6 (¾-cup) servings*

One serving—Calories: 266; Total fat: 15.9 g; Saturated fat: 6.4 g; Cholesterol: 27 mg;
Sodium: 413 mg; Carbohydrates: 21.6 g; Fiber: 1.5 g; Sugar: 4.1 g; Protein: 9 g

## Potato Buffet

2 large baking potatoes

1 teaspoon vegetable oil

Toppings (selected from "Topping Suggestions" following recipe)

1. Preheat oven to 400°F.
2. Wash each potato. Cut each potato in half lengthwise. Brush the outside of each half with the oil.
3. Put one pair of potato halves together (cut sides facing each other). Wrap the potato in foil. Repeat this procedure with the other two halves.
4. Bake the potatoes on the oven rack for 1¼ hours or until tender throughout.
5. While the potatoes bake, set out bowls with the different toppings.
6. Unwrap the foil from the potatoes. Set one-half of a potato on each person's plate. Let people top their potato half with any topping they choose.

**Topping Suggestions**

Chopped chives or green onions

Chili

Cooked ground hamburger mixed with taco sauce

Small cubed pieces of ham (use casein-free ham for dairy-free diets)

Tuna fish salad, warmed in the microwave for a few seconds (do not use canned albacore tuna for dairy-free diets; StarKist Chunk Light Tuna in spring water is casein-free)

Salsa

Shredded Monterey Jack cheese (Vegan Gourmet Monterey Jack Cheese Alternative is gluten- and dairy-free)

Shredded cheddar cheese (Vegan Gourmet Cheddar Cheese Alternative is gluten- and dairy-free)

Broccoli cheddar cheese sauce (Steam the broccoli in the microwave, drain it, sprinkle it with cheese, then microwave it again until the cheese has melted)

*Makes 4 (½-potato) servings*

One serving (no toppings)—Calories: 155; Total fat: 1.3 g; Saturated fat: 0.1 g; Cholesterol: 0 mg; Sodium: 21 mg; Carbohydrates: 32 g; Fiber: 3.4 g; Sugar: 1.6 g; Protein: 3.9 g

## Roasted Potatoes

8 small red-skinned potatoes

3 tablespoons olive oil

¼ teaspoon salt

¼ teaspoon pepper

¾ teaspoon dill weed

1 tablespoon grated Parmesan
cheese (Eat in the Raw Parma!
Vegan Parmesan is gluten- and
dairy-free)

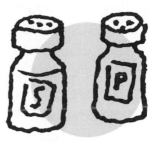

1. Preheat oven to 350°F. Spray a 9″ × 13″ baking pan with gluten-free nonstick spray.
2. Cut the potatoes into ½-inch cubes; put them in a large bowl. Drizzle the olive oil over the potatoes. Stir with a spoon to mix well. Transfer the potatoes to the baking pan.
3. Sprinkle the salt, pepper, dill, and cheese over the top.
4. Cover the pan with foil. Bake the potatoes for 20 minutes. Remove the foil, and then bake for 20 minutes more or until tender.

*Makes 4 (¾-cup) servings*

One serving—Calories: 334; Total fat: 11 g; Saturated fat: 1.7 g; Cholesterol: 1 mg; Sodium: 185 mg; Carbohydrates: 54.3 g; Fiber: 5.8 g; Sugar: 3.4 g; Protein: 7 g

## Potato Pats

1 (15-ounce) can sliced sweet potatoes, well drained

1 teaspoon olive oil

¼ cup milk (use casein-free soy or rice milk for dairy-free diets)

⅛ teaspoon salt

¼ teaspoon cinnamon

¾ teaspoon brown sugar

1¼ cups + 1 cup crushed gluten-free puffed rice cereal (Health
Valley Rice Crunch-Ems! are gluten- and dairy-free)

1. Preheat oven to 350°F. Lightly spray a baking sheet with non-stick spray.
2. Place the sweet potatoes and oil in a medium bowl and mash the potatoes with a fork.
3. Add the milk, salt, cinnamon, and brown sugar. Whip with a fork until all ingredients are smooth.
4. Add 1¼ cups crushed cereal and blend in completely with a rubber spatula.
5. Place the remaining 1 cup of crushed cereal on a dish.
6. Divide the potatoes into eight even sections; form each into a patty, then dip each patty into the crumbs, covering both sides.
7. Lay the patties on the baking sheet. Bake for 15 minutes. Turn patties and continue to bake for another 10 minutes or till lightly browned.

*Makes 4 (2-patty) servings*

One serving—Calories: 164; Total fat: 2.1 g; Saturated fat: 0.6 g; Cholesterol: 1 mg; Sodium: 187 mg; Carbohydrates: 34.5 g; Fiber: 2.9 g; Sugar: 7 g; Protein: 2.6 g

## Glazed Yams

1 (1-pound, 13-ounce) can yams packed in syrup

¼ teaspoon salt

¼ teaspoon pepper

¼ teaspoon cinnamon

Dash ground cloves

¼ cup dark corn syrup

½ cup chopped pecans

½ cup brown sugar

¾ cup crushed gluten-free puffed rice cereal (Perky's Natural Foods Nutty Rice Cereal is gluten- and dairy-free)

¼ cup olive oil

1. Preheat oven to 350°F. Spray an 8″ × 12″ baking pan with nonstick spray.
2. Drain the yams in a sieve over a bowl, reserving ½ cup of the syrup. Place the yams in the baking pan.
3. In a medium bowl, stir together the reserved ½ cup syrup from the yams and the salt, pepper, cinnamon, cloves, and corn syrup. Drizzle this sauce over the yams. Sprinkle the yams with pecans.
4. In a medium bowl, stir together the brown sugar and cereal. Pour the oil over the cereal mixture. Using a fork, mix well to distribute the oil evenly. Sprinkle this mixture over the yams.
5. Bake for 25 minutes.

*Makes 6 (¾-cup) servings*

One serving—Calories: 354; Total fat: 15.9 g; Saturated fat: 1.9 g; Cholesterol: 0 mg; Sodium: 189 mg; Carbohydrates: 53.8 g; Fiber: 3.5 g; Sugar: 26.7 g; Protein: 2.2 g

## Seasoned French Fries

3 tablespoons olive oil

¼ teaspoon salt

⅛ teaspoon pepper

¼ teaspoon garlic powder

2 teaspoons oregano

1 (28-ounce) bag thin frozen french fries

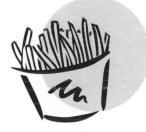

1. Preheat oven to 400°F. Spray a large baking sheet with nonstick spray.
2. In a large bowl, stir together the oil, salt, pepper, garlic powder, and oregano. Add the frozen fries and toss together until the fries are evenly coated.
3. Spread the fries in a single layer on the baking sheet.
4. Bake for 30 minutes or until potatoes are golden brown.

*Makes 8 (3½-ounce) servings*

One serving—Calories: 190; Total fat: 9.6 g; Saturated fat: 1.6 g; Cholesterol: 0 mg; Sodium: 95 mg; Carbohydrates: 24.1 g; Fiber: 2 g; Sugar: 0.2 g; Protein: 2.2 g

## Tomato Potatoes

6 medium red potatoes

1 large tomato

2 green onions

¼ cup olive oil

½ teaspoon salt

¼ teaspoon pepper

1 tablespoon oregano

¼ teaspoon garlic powder

¾ cup minced Monterey Jack cheese (Vegan Gourmet Monterey Jack Cheese Alternative is gluten- and dairy-free)

1 cup water

1 Preheat oven to 350°F. Spray an 8″ × 12″ baking pan with nonstick spray.

2 Chop the potatoes and tomato into 1-inch cubes, then place them in a medium bowl.

3 Thinly slice the green onions and add to the bowl.

4 Add the olive oil, salt, pepper, oregano, garlic powder, cheese, and water. With a spoon, stir until ingredients are blended. Spoon mixture into the baking pan.

5 Bake for 50 minutes or until the potatoes are tender.

*Makes 5 (¾-cup) servings*

One serving—Calories: 355; Total fat: 5.7 g; Saturated fat: 4.8 g; Cholesterol: 15 mg; Sodium: 351 mg; Carbohydrates: 43.3 g; Fiber: 4.8 g; Sugar: 4.1 g; Protein: 9.5 g

# Potato and Green Bean Combo

1 envelope gluten-free dried onion soup mix (Lipton Onion Soup
  Mix is gluten- and dairy-free)

¼ teaspoon pepper

⅓ cup olive oil

1¾ cups milk (use casein-free soy or rice milk for dairy-free diets)

3 large baking potatoes, cut into 1-inch cubes

1 (16-ounce) bag frozen cut green beans, thawed

1 cup crushed corn chips (Fritos Corn Chips are gluten- and dairy-
  free)

1. Preheat oven to 400°F. Spray an 8½″ × 11″ baking pan with nonstick spray.
2. In a large bowl, stir together the soup mix, pepper, oil, and milk.
3. Stir in the potatoes and green beans.
4. Spoon the mixture into the baking pan, then sprinkle the crushed chips on top.
5. Bake for 50 minutes or until the potatoes are tender.

**Note:** Instead of cutting potatoes, you can use 1 (16-ounce) bag frozen hash brown potatoes. Thaw them before adding them to the recipe.

*Makes 6 (1-cup) servings*

One serving—Calories: 445; Total fat: 20.1 g; Saturated fat: 3.8 g; Cholesterol: 7 mg;
Sodium: 684 mg; Carbohydrates: 29 g; Fiber: 5.39 g; Sugar: 7.1 g; Protein: 9.3 g

# Cheesy Tomatoes

3 tablespoons gluten-free cornflake crumbs (Whole Earth
  Corn Flakes are gluten- and dairy-free)

3 tablespoons grated Parmesan cheese (Eat it Raw Parma! Vegan
  Parmesan is gluten- and dairy-free)

⅛ teaspoon garlic powder

⅛ teaspoon Italian seasoning

⅛ teaspoon pepper

2 medium tomatoes

2 teaspoons Italian dressing

1. Preheat oven to 400°F.
2. In a small bowl, stir together the cornflake crumbs, cheese, garlic powder, Italian seasoning, and pepper.
3. Cut each tomato in half.
4. Set the tomato halves, cut side up, in an 8-inch square pan.
5. Drizzle ½ teaspoon Italian dressing on top of each tomato half.
6. Sprinkle each tomato half with the crumb mixture.
7. Bake for 10 minutes or until the crumb mixture is toasted.

*Makes 4 (½-tomato) servings*

One serving—Calories: 42; Total fat: 2.1 g; Saturated fat: 0.8 g; Cholesterol: 3 mg; Sodium: 114 mg; Carbohydrates: 4 g; Fiber: 0.9 g; Sugar: 1.9 g; Protein: 2.1 g

## Baked Italian Vegetables

1 medium zucchini

1 (14½-ounce) can French-cut green beans, drained

1 (14½-ounce) can diced tomatoes, undrained

1 teaspoon minced garlic

1 teaspoon Italian seasoning

¼ teaspoon salt

¼ teaspoon pepper

1. Preheat oven to 375 °F. Spray a 9-inch pie plate with nonstick spray.
2. On a cutting board, cut off both ends of the zucchini and throw away. Cut the zucchini in half lengthwise, then cut each

half into ¼-inch slices. Transfer the zucchini to a medium bowl.

3 Add the drained green beans, diced tomatoes along with their juice, garlic, Italian seasoning, salt, and pepper. Stir to blend well.

4 Spoon mixture into the pie plate. Bake for 35 minutes.

*Makes 4 (1-cup) servings*

One serving—Calories: 56; Total fat: 0.5 g; Saturated fat: 0 g; Cholesterol: 0 mg; Sodium: 568 mg; Carbohydrates: 12.3 g; Fiber: 3.6 g; Sugar: 5.3 g; Protein: 2.5 g

## Cabbage Rice Casserole

1½ cups shredded cabbage (prebagged shredded cabbage or cole slaw can be used)

1 onion, sliced thin

½ cup uncooked instant rice

1¼ cups gluten-free spaghetti sauce (Trader Joe's Organic Tomato Basil Marinara is gluten- and dairy-free)

1 Preheat oven to 350°F. Spray a 1½-quart casserole with non-stick spray.

2 Lay the cabbage in the bottom of the casserole dish.

3 Lay the onion on top of the cabbage.

4 Pour the rice evenly on top of the onion.

5 Spoon the spaghetti sauce on top of the rice.

6 Cover the dish with a lid or foil and bake for 35 minutes.

*Makes 4 (¾-cup) servings*

One serving—Calories: 132; Total fat: 2.3 g; Saturated fat: 0.6 g; Cholesterol: 1 mg; Sodium: 336 mg; Carbohydrates: 24.9 g; Fiber: 2.8 g; Sugar: 9.1 g; Protein: 3 g

# Spanish Rice

1 cup uncooked white or brown rice

1 medium onion, chopped

½ green pepper, chopped

2 tablespoons olive oil

2 cups gluten-free chicken broth
   (Swanson Chicken Broth is
   gluten- and dairy-free)

1 (10-ounce) can diced tomatoes
   with green chilies

¼ teaspoon chili powder

½ teaspoon salt

1 In a medium saucepan, cook the rice, onion, and green pepper in the oil over medium heat, stirring frequently, until the onion is soft.

2 Stir in the broth, tomatoes, chili powder, and salt.

3 Cover the pan, lower the heat to medium-low, and simmer for about 20 minutes or until the liquid has been absorbed.

*Makes 4 (⅔-cup) servings*

One serving—Calories: 256; Total fat: 7.3 g; Saturated fat: 1 g; Cholesterol: 0 mg; Sodium: 1,002 mg; Carbohydrates: 42.7 g; Fiber: 1.4 g; Sugar: 1.8 g; Protein: 4.8 g

# Balsamic Beets

1 (15-ounce) can sliced beets, drained

1 tablespoon balsamic vinegar

1 tablespoon maple syrup

1 tablespoon olive oil

⅛ teaspoon salt

⅛ teaspoon pepper

⅛ teaspoon dried thyme

① Drain the beets in a sieve. Put the drained beets into a medium saucepan.

② In a small bowl, stir together the vinegar, maple syrup, oil, salt, pepper, and thyme. Pour this mixture over the beets.

③ Over medium heat, cook the beets for 5 minutes or until they are glazed. Serve hot.

*Makes 3 (½-cup) servings*

One serving—Calories: 92; Total fat: 4.7 g; Saturated fat: 0.6 g; Cholesterol: 0 mg; Sodium: 289 mg; Carbohydrates: 12.5 g; Fiber: 2.1 g; Sugar: 10.3 g; Protein: 0.9 g

# Really Good Cauliflower

1 (16-ounce) bag frozen cauliflower florets

1 cup mayonnaise

1 tablespoon yellow mustard

8 teaspoons milk (use soy or rice milk for dairy-free diets)

1 cup shredded cheddar cheese (Vegan Gourmet Cheddar Cheese Alternative is gluten- and dairy-free)

① Place the cauliflower florets in a 9-inch glass pie plate. Cover with wax paper and microwave on high for 3 minutes.

② In a small bowl, stir together the mayonnaise, mustard, milk, and cheese. Spoon this mixture over the pieces of cauliflower.

③ Microwave on high for 1 to 2 minutes or until cheese is melted.

*Makes 4 (⅔-cup) servings*

One serving—Calories: 378; Total fat: 29.8 g; Saturated fat: 9.1 g; Cholesterol: 46 mg; Sodium: 667 mg; Carbohydrates: 20.4 g; Fiber: 2.7 g; Sugar: 7 g; Protein: 10.3 g

# Cold Side Dishes

## Egg Bugs

2 eggs
2 cups shredded lettuce
1 cherry tomato
1 teaspoon mayonnaise
1 pitted black olive
2 mini carrots

1. Put uncracked eggs in a small pan. Pour enough water into the pan to cover the eggs. Put the pan on the stove, and bring the water to a boil. Once the water comes to a boil, reduce the heat to medium-high and let the eggs cook in a slow boil for 10 minutes.

2. Remove the hot pan from the stove and pour out the boiling water. Set the pan in the sink, and let cold running water fill the pan. (This helps stop the eggs from cooking more.) Remove the eggs from the pan. Peel the eggs under cold running water.

3. Cut a thin slice from one side of each egg (so the eggs will lie flat without rolling over). Lay 1 cup of lettuce on each of two dishes. Place one egg, cut side down, on top of the lettuce on each dish.

4. Cut the tomato in half. Put a dab of mayonnaise on the cut side of one of the tomato halves, and stick that side to the pointed end of the egg (for the head of your bug). Put a dab of mayonnaise on the cut side of the second tomato half and stick it to the pointed end of the second egg.

5. Cut four slices from the olive. Use mayonnaise to stick two olive "eyes" to each tomato head. With a toothpick, use mayonnaise to draw a mouth on the tomato "heads."

6. Shred the carrots. Use mayonnaise to stick the carrot "hair" to the tops of the tomato "heads."

*Makes 2 egg bugs*

One egg bug—Calories: 105; Total fat: 6.6 g; Saturated fat: 1.8 g; Cholesterol: 213 mg; Sodium: 117 mg; Carbohydrates: 4.4 g; Fiber: 1.3 g; Sugar: 2.7 g; Protein: 7.2 g

# Potato Salad

2 cans (14½ ounces each) whole potatoes, drained and cut into
    ½-inch cubes

½ small onion, chopped

⅓ cup chopped green pepper

2 hard-boiled eggs, peeled and chopped

¼ cup mayonnaise

¾ teaspoon yellow mustard

¼ teaspoon salt

¼ teaspoon black pepper

⅛ teaspoon paprika

1 Put the potatoes, onion, green pepper, and eggs into a medium bowl.

2 In a small bowl, stir together the mayonnaise, mustard, salt, and black pepper. When blended, spoon this mixture over the potato mixture and blend well.

3 Spoon the mixture into a serving bowl and sprinkle the top with paprika. Cover and refrigerate for several hours to allow flavors to blend.

*Makes 6 (1-cup) servings*

One serving—Calories: 99; Total fat: 5.2 g; Saturated fat: 1.1 g; Cholesterol: 73.2 mg; Sodium: 306 mg; Carbohydrates: 10.4 g; Fiber: 1 g; Sugar: 1.2 g; Protein: 3.1 g

# Cole Slaw

¾ cup mayonnaise

¼ cup apple cider vinegar

1½ tablespoons sugar

½ teaspoon garlic powder

½ teaspoon salt

½ teaspoon pepper

½ teaspoon paprika

1 (8-ounce) bag shredded
   cabbage with shredded
   carrots

1 small onion, shredded

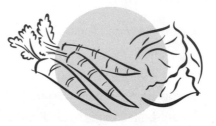

1. In a large bowl, stir together the mayonnaise, vinegar, sugar, garlic powder, salt, pepper, and paprika until smooth.
2. Add the cabbage mix and onion. Stir until blended.
3. Cover the bowl with plastic wrap. Refrigerate for several hours to blend flavors.

*Makes 6 (¾-cup) servings*

One serving—Calories: 117; Total fat: 5.6 g; Saturated fat: 0.9 g; Cholesterol: 7 mg; Sodium: 404 mg; Carbohydrates: 14.7 g; Fiber: 1.6 g; Sugar: 6.7 g; Protein: 1.1 g

# Mixed Bean Salad

1 (16-ounce) can garbanzo beans

1 (16-ounce) can black beans

1 (16-ounce) can kidney beans

1 (16-ounce) can Great Northern beans

½ green pepper, chopped fine

1 onion, chopped fine

⅓ cup olive oil

3 tablespoons balsamic vinegar

¼ teaspoon salt

¼ teaspoon black pepper

¼ teaspoon garlic powder

1 teaspoon dried dill weed

¼ teaspoon mint flakes

¼ teaspoon ground oregano

**1** Put all of the beans in a large colander. Rinse well under cold running water, then drain. Transfer the beans to a large bowl. Stir in the green pepper and onion.

**2** In a small bowl, whisk together the olive oil, vinegar, salt, black pepper, garlic powder, dill, mint, and oregano. Pour the dressing over the bean mixture. Stir well to evenly coat the beans. Cover and refrigerate several hours to let the flavors blend.

*Makes 10 (¾-cup) servings*

One serving—Calories: 175; Total fat: 7.8 g; Saturated fat: 11.1 g; Cholesterol: 0 mg; Sodium: 301 mg; Carbohydrates: 20.9 g; Fiber: 5.7 g; Sugar: 1.8 g; Protein: 6.1 g

## Italian Marinated Salad

1 medium cucumber, sliced into ¼-inch slices

2 medium tomatoes, sliced into ¼-inch slices

¼ pound mozzarella cheese, cut into thin slices (Vegan Gourmet Mozzarella Cheese Alternative is gluten- and dairy-free)

8 slices deli ham, each slice cut into quarters

¼ red onion, sliced very thin

¼ teaspoon basil

¼ teaspoon garlic powder

⅛ teaspoon black pepper

¼ teaspoon sugar

Dash red pepper flakes

2 tablespoons balsamic vinegar

3 tablespoons olive oil

1 Lay cucumber, tomato, cheese, ham, and onion slices, slightly overlapping, in a circle on each of four salad plates, dividing evenly.

2 In a small bowl, whisk together the basil, garlic powder, black pepper, sugar, red pepper flakes, vinegar, and olive oil.

3 Drizzle the dressing over the salads.

*Makes 4 (¾-cup) servings*

One serving—Calories: 251; Total fat: 17 g; Saturated fat: 5 g; Cholesterol: 46 mg; Sodium: 840 mg; Carbohydrates: 9 g; Fiber: 1.4 g; Sugar: 5.2 g; Protein: 16.2 g

## Strawberry Spinach Salad

1 (8-ounce) bag baby spinach leaves

8 fresh strawberries

½ cup pecans in small pieces

¼ cup shelled sunflower seeds

¼ cup olive oil

1 tablespoon balsamic vinegar

2 tablespoons raspberry jam

¼ teaspoon pepper

1 Place the spinach leaves onto six salad plates, dividing evenly.

2 Cut the leaves off the top of the strawberries. Wash the strawberries, and then pat them dry. Slice each strawberry. Divide the strawberry slices evenly among the salad plates.

3 Sprinkle each salad with pecans and sunflower seeds.

4 In a small bowl, whisk together the olive oil, vinegar, jam, and pepper. Drizzle the salad dressing over the salads.

*Makes 6 (1-cup) servings*

One serving—Calories: 214; Total fat: 18.9 g; Saturated fat: 2.2 g; Cholesterol: 0 mg; Sodium: 4 mg; Carbohydrates: 10.4 g; Fiber: 2.9 g; Sugar: 5 g; Protein: 3.3 g

# Tuna Pasta Salad

This pasta salad is delicious served while the macaroni is still warm, or you can cover the salad, refrigerate it for several hours, and serve it cold.

1 (8-ounce) can cut green beans, drained

1 onion, chopped

1 tablespoon dried parsley

10 cherry tomatoes, cut in half

1 clove garlic, minced

¼ cup olive oil

1 tablespoon cider vinegar

1 teaspoon brown mustard

¼ teaspoon salt

¼ teaspoon pepper

1 teaspoon Italian seasoning

1 (6½-ounce) can water-packed tuna, drained (use casein-free canned tuna for dairy-free diets)

1 cup gluten-free corkscrew or elbow macaroni

1 In a large bowl, use a large spoon to mix together the green beans, onion, dried parsley, tomatoes, garlic, oil, vinegar, mustard, salt, pepper, Italian seasoning, and tuna fish.

2 Cook the macaroni in boiling water according to package directions. Rinse the macaroni under cold running water, then drain in a colander.

3 Toss the warm macaroni with the tuna mixture.

*Makes 5 (1-cup) servings*

One serving—Calories: 337; Total fat: 11.6 g; Saturated fat: 1.7 g; Cholesterol: 11 mg; Sodium: 481 mg; Carbohydrates: 44.4 g; Fiber: 3 g; Sugar: 2.3 g; Protein: 15.9 g

## Chicken Salad

¼ small onion, chopped fine

1 rib celery, sliced thin

¼ green pepper, chopped fine

2 tablespoons chopped fresh parsley

1 (6-ounce) cooked chicken breast,
  cut into small cubes

½ cup drained pineapple tidbits

⅛ teaspoon salt

⅛ teaspoon black pepper

¼ cup mayonnaise

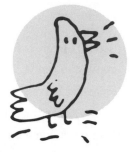

1. Place the onion, celery, green pepper, parsley, and chicken cubes in a large bowl.
2. Add the pineapple, salt, black pepper, and mayonnaise. Stir well until combined.
3. Cover the bowl with a piece of plastic wrap. Chill the salad in the refrigerator for an hour to let the flavors blend.

*Makes 2 (1-cup) servings*

One serving—Calories: 278; Total fat: 12.9 g; Saturated fat: 2.2 g; Cholesterol: 83 mg; Sodium: 663 mg; Carbohydrates: 16.5 g; Fiber: 1.5 g; Sugar: 9.4 g; Protein: 25.7 g

## Cranberry Mold

1 (3-ounce) box strawberry gelatin

1 cup boiling water

1 (16-ounce) can whole-berry cranberry sauce

½ cup peeled and finely chopped apple

½ cup finely chopped celery

1. Pour the gelatin into a medium bowl. Carefully add the boiling water. Stir until the gelatin is completely dissolved.
2. In a small bowl, break up the cranberry sauce with a fork, then add it to the gelatin mixture. Stir until the cranberry sauce is dissolved.

3 Refrigerate the gelatin mixture until it is almost gelled, about 1½ hours.

4 Fold in the apples and celery.

5 Pour the mixture into a mold pan (or keep it in the mixing bowl). Chill until the gelatin is set, about 3 hours.

*Makes 4 (1-cup) servings*

One serving—Calories: 215; Total fat: 0.2 g; Saturated fat: 0 g; Cholesterol: 0 mg; Sodium: 133 mg; Carbohydrates: 53.7 g; Fiber: 1.1 g; Sugar: 51.4 g; Protein: 1.9 g

## Cranberry Cherry Mold

1 (16-ounce) can jellied cranberry sauce
1 (16½-ounce) can pitted dark sweet cherries, undrained
1 (10½-ounce) can crushed pineapple, undrained
1 (6-ounce) box cherry gelatin
1 cup chopped walnuts

1 Melt the cranberry sauce in a medium saucepan over low heat.

2 Drain the juice from the cherries into a 2-cup measuring cup and set aside.

3 Cut the cherries into quarters. Stir them into the melted cranberry sauce.

4 Stir in the pineapple, including the juice from the can.

5 Remove the pan from the heat.

6 Add enough water to the reserved cherry juice to make 2 cups. Pour the juice and water into a small saucepan. Bring the cherry juice mixture to a boil on the stove.

7 Put the gelatin into a medium bowl.

8 Carefully pour the boiling cherry mixture over the gelatin. Stir until the gelatin is completely dissolved.

9 Stir in the cranberry mixture and the nuts.

10 Pour the gelatin mixture into a mold or a 9″ × 13″ baking pan. Refrigerate until firm, about 5 hours.

*Makes 18 (3″ × 2″) servings*

One serving—Calories: 146; Total fat: 4.3 g; Saturated fat: 0.4 g; Cholesterol: 0 mg; Sodium: 52 mg; Carbohydrates: 26.4 g; Fiber: 1.2 g; Sugar: 23.5 g; Protein: 2 g

## No-Cook Applesauce

3 apples, any variety

2 tablespoons freshly squeezed lemon juice

¼ cup sugar

¼ teaspoon cinnamon

1  Peel and core the apples, removing all seeds. Chop the apples into small pieces. Put the apple pieces into a blender.

2  Add the lemon juice, sugar, and cinnamon to the blender.

3  Puree the apple mixture until smooth, stopping the machine to scrape down the sides frequently. Total puree time is about 1 minute.

*Makes 4 (¾-cup) servings*

One serving—Calories: 85; Total fat: 0.5 g; Saturated fat: 0 g; Cholesterol: 0 mg; Sodium: 0 mg; Carbohydrates: 22 g; Fiber: 2.7 g; Sugar: 19 g; Protein: 0.2 g

# 7

# Desserts

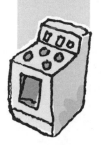

## Paintbrush Cookies

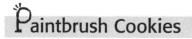

Gluten-free sugar cookie dough (make dairy-free dough for a dairy-free diet)

3 egg yolks

3 tablespoons water

3 different food colorings

Colored gluten-free sprinkles (optional)

1. Make one recipe of your favorite sugar cookie dough. Preheat oven according to cookie dough instructions.
2. Lightly spray a baking sheet with nonstick spray.
3. Roll out the cookie dough, ½ inch thick. Cut with cookie cutters, then carefully place cookies on the baking sheet.
4. Place an egg yolk in each of three small cups. Add 1 tablespoon of water to each cup. Using a fork, mix the water and egg yolk in each cup.
5. Add a drop of food coloring to each cup; stir to blend.
6. With a thin, clean paintbrush, use the colored egg yolks to "paint" the top of the cookies, making beautiful designs and

pictures. Sprinkle the tops of the cookies with colored sprinkles if you are using them.

7 Bake your creations following the cookie recipe directions.

*Makes 3 (⅓-cup) servings of "paint"*

One serving—Calories: 54; Total fat: 4.5 g; Saturated fat: 1.6 g; Cholesterol: 210 mg; Sodium: 8 mg; Carbohydrates: 0.6 g; Fiber: 0 g; Sugar: 0.1 g; Protein: 2.7 g

## Rocky Road Bars

½ cup butter (use dairy-free margarine for dairy-free diets)

½ cup granulated sugar

½ cup brown sugar

½ cup peanut butter

2½ teaspoons vanilla

2 eggs

1½ cups gluten-free flour mixture (See the Gluten-Free Flour Mixtures on page 16)

1 cup chopped unsalted peanuts

1 cup coarsely chopped dark chocolate

2 cups miniature marshmallows (Sweet & Sara brand marshmallows are gluten- and dairy-free)

1 Preheat oven to 375°F. Spray a 9″ × 13″ baking pan with non-stick spray.

2 Put the butter in a glass measuring cup. Place it in the microwave on full power for 20 seconds or until the butter has melted.

3 In a large bowl, stir together the melted butter, granulated and brown sugars, peanut butter, vanilla, and eggs.

4 Stir in the flour mixture until well combined. Press the dough into the pan. Bake for 10 minutes.

5 Remove the hot pan from the oven. Sprinkle the peanuts over the crust, then the chocolate pieces, and finally the marshmallows.

6. Put the pan back in the oven to bake for another 8 to 10 minutes, until marshmallows puff and get lightly browned. Cool thoroughly before cutting. Cut into 3″ × 2″ bars.

*Makes 18 (3″ × 2″) bars*

One bar—Calories: 302; Total fat: 17.5 g; Saturated fat: 6.3 g; Cholesterol: 38 mg; Sodium: 86 mg; Carbohydrates: 34.6 g; Fiber: 2.3 g; Sugar: 19.3 g; Protein: 6.93 g

## Toffee Squares

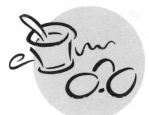

1 cup butter, melted (use stick dairy-free margarine
    for dairy-free diets)
1 cup brown sugar
2 eggs
1½ teaspoons vanilla
2 cups gluten-free flour
    mixture (See the Gluten-
    Free Flour Mixtures on
    page 16)
¾ cup finely chopped dark chocolate
½ cup chopped walnuts

1. Preheat oven to 350°F. Spray a 9″ × 13″ baking pan with nonstick spray.
2. Put the butter, brown sugar, eggs, and vanilla in a large bowl. Mix with a whisk until smooth.
3. Stir in the flour mixture with a rubber spatula until it is completely blended.
4. Spread the dough on the bottom of the baking pan. Bake for 15 minutes.
5. Remove the pan from the oven and set it on a cooling rack, on top of the stove, on a cutting board, or on pot holders. Sprinkle the chocolate pieces on top of the dough and bake for another 2 minutes.

6  Using the back of a small spoon, spread the melted chocolate pieces to form an even coating on top.

7  Sprinkle the nuts on top of the chocolate. Cool before cutting into 30 bars.

*Makes 30 (3″ × 1″) bars*

One bar—Calories: 161; Total fat: 9.7 g; Saturated fat: 5.2 g; Cholesterol: 31 mg; Sodium: 53 mg; Carbohydrates: 18.4 g; Fiber: 1 g; Sugar: 10.3 g; Protein: 1.4 g

## Granola Bars

⅔ cup vegetable oil

½ cup brown sugar

½ cup light corn syrup

2 teaspoons vanilla

¼ cup gluten-free flour mixture (See the Gluten-Free Flour Mixtures on page 16)

3 cups pure oats

½ cup shredded coconut

½ cup sunflower seeds

½ cup sesame seeds

½ cup chopped pecans

⅓ cup chopped dark chocolate

⅓ cup raisins

1  Preheat oven to 350 °F. Spray a 9″ × 13″ pan well with nonstick spray.

2  In a large bowl, use a rubber spatula to blend the oil, brown sugar, corn syrup, and vanilla.

3  Stir in the flour mixture and oats until blended.

4  Add the coconut, sunflower seeds, sesame seeds, pecans, chocolate, and raisins. Stir until evenly blended.

5  Spoon mixture into the baking pan. Smooth top with wet fingers. Bake for 30 minutes or until top is golden. Allow granola mixture to cool completely before cutting into bars.

*Makes 48 (2¼" × 1") bars*

One bar—Calories: 125; Total fat: 6.7 g; Saturated fat: 1.1 g; Cholesterol: 0 mg;
Sodium: 6.9 mg; Carbohydrates: 14.5 g; Fiber: 4 g; Sugar: 2.8 g; Protein: 2.4 g

## Applesauce Bars

⅓ cup vegetable oil

⅔ cup applesauce

2 eggs

1 teaspoon vanilla

2 teaspoons mayonnaise

1 cup brown sugar

2¼ cups gluten-free flour mixture (See the Gluten-Free Flour
  Mixtures on page 16)

1 tablespoon baking powder

1½ teaspoons baking soda

½ teaspoon salt

1 teaspoon cinnamon

1 cup raisins

¾ cup chopped walnuts

Powdered sugar (optional)

1. Preheat oven to 350°F. Spray a 9" × 13" baking pan with non-stick spray.

2. In a large bowl, mix the oil, applesauce, eggs, vanilla, and mayonnaise with a whisk, and then whisk in the brown sugar.

3. Add the flour mixture, baking powder, baking soda, salt, and cinnamon to the applesauce mixture. With a rubber spatula, stir the dough until blended.

4. Stir in the raisins and walnuts.

5. Spread the batter in the baking pan. Smooth the top of the batter with a wet rubber spatula.

6. Bake the batter for 20 minutes or until a toothpick inserted in the center comes out clean.

7. When the pastry has cooled, sift powdered sugar over the top, if desired. Cut into 30 bars.

*Makes 30 (3" × 1") bars*

One bar—Calories: 129; Total fat: 4.9 g; Saturated fat: 0.5 g; Cholesterol: 14 mg; Sodium: 148 mg; Carbohydrates: 20.5 g; Fiber: 0.9 g; Sugar: 10.6 g; Protein: 1.4 g

## Best-Ever Chocolate Cookies

¾ cup + ¾ cup coarsely chopped dark chocolate

2 eggs

3 tablespoons vegetable oil

2 teaspoons vanilla

¾ cup brown sugar

¾ cup gluten-free flour mixture
   (See the Gluten-Free Flour
   Mixtures on page 16)

¾ teaspoon baking powder

1 cup chopped walnuts

1. Preheat oven to 350°F.

2. Put ¾ cup of the chocolate pieces into a large microwave-safe bowl. Microwave on high for 30 seconds. Stir the chocolate, and then continue to microwave until just melted (for about another 15 seconds).

3. Whisk in the eggs, oil, vanilla, and brown sugar until blended.

4. Add the flour mixture and baking powder. Stir mixture until well blended.

5. Stir in the remaining ¾ cup chocolate pieces and the walnuts.

6. Drop the batter by rounded tablespoonfuls onto an ungreased cookie sheet.

7 Bake for 12 minutes or until the cookies are puffed and no imprint is left when you touch the top of a cookie very lightly. Do not let the cookies brown too much on the bottom or the cookies will be overbaked. Let the cookies cool on a wire rack.

*Makes 48 cookies*

One cookie—Calories: 84; Total fat: 5.1 g; Saturated fat: 1.7 g; Cholesterol: 9.7 mg; Sodium: 13 mg; Carbohydrates: 10.1 g; Fiber: 0.8 g; Sugar: 7.2 g; Protein: 1.1 g

## oconut Nut Bars

1 cup gluten-free flour mixture (See the Gluten-Free Flour Mixtures on page 16)

½ cup butter (use stick dairy-free margarine for dairy-free diets)

1 teaspoon vanilla

¼ cup granulated sugar

2 eggs

1½ cups brown sugar

1 cup chopped walnuts

½ cup shredded coconut

1 Preheat oven to 350°F. Lightly spray a 9-inch square pan with nonstick spray.

2 Spoon the flour mixture into a medium bowl.

3 With the back of a fork, blend in the butter and the vanilla. Add the granulated sugar, continuing to blend with the fork until the butter is in teeny pieces.

4 Pat the pastry into the bottom of the pan.

5 In a medium bowl, whisk the eggs until frothy and then whisk in the brown sugar.

6 Stir in the walnuts and coconut.

7 Spoon the egg mixture over the pastry.

8 Bake for 25 minutes or until the top is golden. Cool the baked mixture in the pan. When cooled, cut into 36 squares.

*Makes 36 (1½″ × 1½″) squares*

One square—Calories: 107; Total fat: 5.3 g; Saturated fat: 2.2 g; Cholesterol: 19 mg; Sodium: 28.4 mg; Carbohydrates: 14 g; Fiber: 0.4 g; Sugar: 10.8 g; Protein: 1.1 g

## Super Simple S'Mores

> 8 gluten-free cookies (your favorite flavor, store-bought or
> home-baked)
> 1 (1.45-ounce) dark chocolate candy bar (Amanda's Own
> Confections offers gluten- and dairy-free chocolate bars)
> 4 large marshmallows (AllerEnergy makes dairy-free
> marshmallows)

1. Place four of the cookies on a microwave-safe dish with the top side down. Top each cookie with one-fourth of the candy bar and then 1 marshmallow.
2. Microwave on medium power for 10 to 20 seconds or until the marshmallows expand.
3. Remove the dish from the microwave and top each marshmallow with a cookie.

*Makes 4 servings*

One serving (made with chocolate chip cookies)—Calories: 308; Total fat: 17 g; Saturated fat: 10 g; Cholesterol: 21 mg; Sodium: 149 mg; Carbohydrates: 40.1 g; Fiber: 1.7 g; Sugar: 17.4 g; Protein: 1.6 g

## Raspberry Squares

**Crust**

> 1 cup gluten-free flour mixture (See the Gluten-Free Flour Mixtures
> on page 16)
> 2 teaspoons baking powder
> 1 tablespoon sugar
> ½ cup butter, softened (use stick dairy-free margarine for dairy-free
> diets)

2 eggs

1 tablespoon milk

**Filling**

½ cup raspberry jam

1 teaspoon almond extract

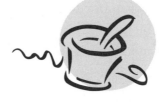

**Topping**

1 egg

¼ cup butter, melted (use dairy-free margarine for dairy-free diets)

1 teaspoon vanilla

1 cup sugar

2 cups shredded coconut

1. Preheat oven to 350°F. Lightly spray a 9-inch square pan with nonstick spray.

2. To make the crust, whisk together the flour mixture and baking powder in a medium bowl. With the back of a fork, work the 1 tablespoon sugar and ½ cup butter into the flour mixture until it is like small crumbs. In a small bowl, whisk 2 eggs until frothy. Add the eggs and milk to the flour mixture, mixing well until blended.

3. With lightly floured hands, pat the pastry into the bottom of the baking pan.

4. To make the filling, stir together the raspberry jam and almond extract in a small bowl. Spread the filling over the pastry.

5. To make the topping, whisk together 1 egg, melted butter, and vanilla in a medium bowl. Stir 1 cup sugar into the egg mixture. Stir in the coconut. With the back of a spoon, spread the topping evenly over the raspberry layer.

6. Bake for 30 minutes or until the topping is golden brown. Cool the pastry in the pan. Cut into 24 pieces.

*Makes 24 (2¼″ × 1½″) squares*

One square—Calories: 166; Total fat: 8.4 g; Saturated fat: 0.3 g; Cholesterol: 42 mg; Sodium: 103 mg; Carbohydrates: 21.8 g; Fiber: 1 g; Sugar: 14.8 g; Protein: 1.3 g

**Note:** Dairy-free margarine is available in sticks (like butter) and in tubs. For many dessert recipes, it is important to use the stick margarine because the mixture that comes in tubs contains too much water. The high water content in the tubs can affect the outcome of your dessert.

## Candy Bar Cookies

1 cup peanut butter

1 cup light corn syrup

½ cup chopped dark chocolate

⅓ cup brown sugar

1 teaspoon vanilla

¾ cup chopped dry-roasted peanuts

½ cup sesame seeds

½ cup sunflower seeds

1½ cups crushed gluten-free puffed rice cereal (Arrowhead Mills makes gluten- and dairy-free puffed rice cereal)

1. Spray a 9-inch square pan with nonstick spray.
2. In a medium saucepan, stir together the peanut butter, corn syrup, chocolate, and brown sugar. Simmer the mixture over medium heat, stirring constantly with a wooden spoon until the chocolate has melted (about 5 minutes).
3. Stir in the vanilla, and then stir in the peanuts, sesame seeds, and sunflower seeds.
4. Stir in the cereal until well blended. Keep in mind that the mixture will be thick.
5. Press the mixture into the baking pan. With damp hands, press down gently and smooth the top so it is level. Let the mixture set at room temperature for 1 hour before cutting into bars. Do not refrigerate the bars or they will become too hard.

*Makes 36 (1½" × 1½") squares*

One square—Calories: 135; Total fat: 7.9 g; Saturated fat: 1.8 g; Cholesterol: 0.04 mg; Sodium: 21 mg; Carbohydrates: 15.6 g; Fiber: 1.5 g; Sugar: 7 g; Protein: 3.2 g

# No-Bake Delights

5 tablespoons butter, melted (use dairy-free margarine for dairy-free diets)

½ cup milk (use casein-free vanilla soy, rice, or almond milk for dairy-free diets)

1 cup sugar

6 tablespoons unsweetened cocoa

1½ tablespoons vanilla

1 cup chopped walnuts

1 cup shredded coconut

1 cup crumbled gluten-free cookies (Shortcake Rings by Glutano and Shortcake Dreams by Glutino are gluten- and dairy-free)

5 tablespoons chopped dark chocolate

1. Line a baking sheet with wax paper.
2. In a medium, microwave-safe bowl, stir together the butter, milk, sugar, and cocoa. Place the bowl in the microwave and cook for 3 minutes, stirring after each minute. Stir in the vanilla, walnuts, coconut, and cookie crumbs. Stir in the dark chocolate.
3. Drop tablespoonfuls of the mixture onto the wax paper. Cover the pan with foil and refrigerate for 3 hours to set cookies.

*Makes 40 cookies*

One cookie—Calories: 86; Total fat: 5.2 g; Saturated fat: 2.3 g; Cholesterol: 4 mg; Sodium: 25 mg; Carbohydrates: 10.1 g; Fiber: 0.8 g; Sugar: 7.5 g; Protein: 1 g

# Lemon Sugar Cookies

2 eggs

½ cup vegetable oil

1⅔ cups + 2 tablespoons sugar

1 tablespoon milk (use casein-free vanilla soy or rice milk)

2 teaspoons lemon juice

2½ teaspoons vanilla

1 teaspoon lemon extract

2 cups gluten-free flour mixture (See the Gluten-Free Flour
    Mixtures on page 16)

2 teaspoons baking powder

¼ teaspoon salt

½ teaspoon cinnamon

1. Preheat oven to 350 °F. Lightly spray a baking sheet with non-stick spray.

2. Break eggs into a large bowl. Using a wire whisk, whip eggs until frothy.

3. Add the oil, 1⅔ cups sugar, milk, lemon juice, vanilla, and lemon extract. Whisk together till blended.

4. Add the flour mixture, baking powder, salt, and cinnamon. Using a rubber spatula, stir in the dry ingredients until thoroughly blended.

5. With wet hands, take tablespoonfuls of dough and roll each into a ball about the size of a large walnut, then place on the baking sheet.

6. With the bottom of a wet glass, slightly flatten each cookie. Sprinkle the tops of the cookies with the remaining 2 tablespoons sugar.

7. Bake for 12 to 15 minutes or until no imprint remains when center of cookie is lightly touched. Let cookies set on baking pan for 1 minute before removing them to a cooling rack.

**Note:** To make cutout cookies, cover and refrigerate the dough for one hour. Roll the cookie dough out on a flat surface that has been sprinkled with powdered sugar.

*Makes 58 cookies*

One cookie—Calories: 61; Total fat: 2.1 g; Saturated fat: 0.3 g; Cholesterol: 7 mg; Sodium: 25 mg; Carbohydrates: 10 g; Fiber: 6.3 g; Sugar: 0.07 g; Protein: 0.4 g

## Banana Biscotti

1 egg

2 tablespoons + 2 teaspoons vegetable oil

¼ cup milk (use casein-free vanilla soy or rice milk for dairy-free diets)

1½ teaspoons vanilla

½ cup + 2 tablespoons sugar

2 medium bananas

1 cup gluten-free flour mixture (See the Gluten-Free Flour Mixtures on page 16)

¼ teaspoon salt

⅓ cup coarsely chopped walnuts

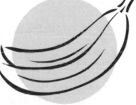

1. Preheat oven to 350°F. Spray a 9-inch square baking pan with nonstick spray.
2. In a medium bowl, whisk the egg until frothy. Add the oil, milk, and vanilla and whisk again. Then add the sugar and whisk until ingredients are blended.
3. In a small bowl, mash the bananas with the back of a fork, and then stir them into the egg mixture.
4. Add the flour and salt, stirring well with a rubber spatula.
5. Stir in the walnuts.
6. Spoon batter into the baking pan. Using a wet spatula, smooth out the top of the batter.

7. Bake for 45 minutes or until the top is golden and a toothpick inserted in the center comes out clean. Remove pan from oven and let it cool.

8. Cut the cake down the center. Turn the pan and cut the cake into ¾-inch slices. Remove the slices and lay them down on a baking sheet.

9. Bake the slices for 12 minutes, and then turn them over and bake for 10 minutes more. Watch them closely. The slices should be barely golden and still just a little soft. Don't over-bake them or they will become too hard once they cool. Cool slices, then store in a self-seal plastic bag.

*Makes 24 biscotti*

One biscotto—Calories: 79; Total fat: 24.5 g; Saturated fat: 0.3 g; Cholesterol: 9 mg; Sodium: 28 mg; Carbohydrates: 12.4 g; Fiber: 0.6 g; Sugar: 6.7 g; Protein: 0.9 g

## Dessert Pizzas

⅔ cup gluten-free flour mixture (See the Gluten-Free Flour Mixtures on page 16)

⅓ cup unsweetened cocoa

½ teaspoon baking powder

⅛ teaspoon salt

¾ cup sugar

1 egg

2 teaspoons vanilla

6 tablespoons butter, melted (use dairy-free stick margarine for dairy-free diets)

¾ cup chopped dark chocolate

Toppings (see "Topping Suggestions" following recipe)

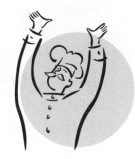

1. Preheat oven to 350°F. Spray two 9-inch round cake pans with a nonstick spray.

2. In a medium bowl, whisk together the flour mixture, cocoa, baking powder, salt, and sugar until blended.

③ In a small bowl, whisk the egg. Add the vanilla and cooled, melted butter and whisk again until blended. With a rubber spatula, stir this mixture into the flour mix until completely blended and the dough leaves the side of the bowl.

④ Pat half of the dough into each of the two cake pans. Bake for 18 to 20 minutes or until a toothpick inserted in the center comes out clean.

⑤ Run a knife around the edge of the cakes. Invert the cakes onto serving plates. Immediately sprinkle the tops of the cakes with the chocolate and let it stand for 5 minutes to melt.

⑥ With the back of a spoon, spread the chocolate over the cakes.

⑦ Sprinkle your favorite toppings over your "pizza." Let pizza cool to room temperature, then cut each cake into 8 wedges.

**Note:** If you love peanut butter, drop dollops of peanut butter (¼ cup total per pizza) on top of the hot pizza base when you add the dark chocolate bits. Let this rest for 5 minutes to melt both items and then, using the back of a small spoon, spread the chocolate-peanut butter mixture over the top of the pizzas.

### Topping Suggestions

  Chopped walnuts or pecans

  Chopped or sliced fresh strawberries

  Chopped maraschino cherries

  Coconut

  Crumbled gluten-free cookies

  Miniature marshmallows

  Raisins

*Makes 16 wedges*

One wedge (without added toppings)—Calories: 158; Total fat: 8.5 g; Saturated fat: 5.1 g; Cholesterol: 26 mg; Sodium: 70 mg; Carbohydrates: 21.9 g; Fiber: 1.7 g; Sugar: 15.2 g; Protein: 1.6 g

# Mock Mounds Bar Treats

1 cup flaked coconut

¾ tablespoon butter, softened (use dairy-free margarine for dairy-free diets)

2 teaspoons milk (use casein-free vanilla soy or rice milk for dairy-free diets)

1½ tablespoons vegetable oil

½ cup chopped dark chocolate

1. In a small bowl, using a fork, stir together the coconut, butter, and milk until the mixture holds together. It may be necessary to add an additional ½ teaspoon or more of milk, depending on how moist the coconut is.
2. Form the coconut mixture into 1-inch balls. Place the balls on a dish or baking sheet that has been lined with wax paper.
3. Put the oil and chocolate in a microwave-safe bowl. Cook on medium power, stirring every 30 seconds, until the chocolate has melted.
4. Spoon the chocolate mixture over the coconut balls, covering the tops completely. Refrigerate about 1 hour to harden the chocolate coating. Store in the refrigerator in a tightly covered plastic container.

*Makes 15 treats*

One treat—Calories: 82; Total fat: 6.1 g; Saturated fat: 3.5 g; Cholesterol: 2 mg; Sodium: 24 mg; Carbohydrates: 7.9 g; Fiber: 1.2 g; Sugar: 6.2 g; Protein: 0.6 g

# Pumpkin Snack Cake

1 egg

1 cup sugar

¼ cup vegetable oil

¾ cup canned pumpkin

1½ teaspoons vanilla

1¼ cups gluten-free flour blend (See the Gluten-Free Flour Mixtures on page 16)

2½ teaspoons baking powder

1 teaspoon baking soda

2 teaspoons cinnamon

1 teaspoon nutmeg

¼ teaspoon salt

¾ cup chopped dark chocolate

¾ cup chopped pecans

1. Preheat oven to 350°F. Spray an 8″ × 11″ baking pan with a nonstick spray.
2. In a medium bowl, whisk the egg until frothy. Add the sugar, oil, pumpkin, and vanilla and continue to whisk until blended.
3. With a rubber spatula, stir in the flour mixture, baking powder, baking soda, cinnamon, nutmeg, and salt until completely blended.
4. Stir in the chocolate pieces and pecans.
5. Spoon the batter into the baking pan. Use a wet rubber spatula to smooth the top. Bake for 25 minutes or until a toothpick inserted in the center comes out clean.

*Makes 12 (2¾″ × 2⅔″) servings*

One serving—Calories: 290; Total fat: 15 g; Saturated fat: 3.8 g; Cholesterol: 19 mg; Sodium: 242 mg; Carbohydrates: 40.1 g; Fiber: 3.1 g; Sugar: 25.2 g; Protein: 2.6 g

## Orange Cake

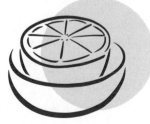

2 eggs

½ cup granulated sugar

½ cup vegetable oil

½ cup orange juice

1 tablespoon grated orange zest

1 teaspoon vanilla

1¼ cups gluten-free flour mixture (See the Gluten-Free Flour
    Mixtures on page 16)
1 tablespoon baking powder
½ teaspoon salt
Powdered sugar

1. Preheat oven to 350°F. Spray a 9-inch square pan with non-stick spray.
2. Whisk the eggs in a medium bowl until frothy.
3. Add the granulated sugar, oil, orange juice, orange zest, and vanilla and whisk until blended.
4. With a rubber spatula, stir in the flour mixture, baking powder, and salt until batter is smooth.
5. Pour the batter into the baking pan. Bake for 20 minutes or until a toothpick inserted in the center comes out clean.
6. When the cake has cooled, sift powdered sugar over the top of the cake.

*Makes 9 (3-inch square) servings*

One serving—Calories: 243; Total fat: 13.7 g; Saturated fat: 2.1 g; Cholesterol: 47 mg; Sodium: 266 mg; Carbohydrates: 28.1 g; Fiber: 0.9 g; Sugar: 11.3 g; Protein: 2.1 g

## 3-Minute Cake

⅓ cup gluten-free flour mixture (See the Gluten-Free Flour Mixtures
    on page 16)
⅓ cup sugar
¼ teaspoon baking powder
Dash of salt
1 tablespoon + 1 teaspoon unsweetened cocoa
1 egg
1 tablespoon + 2 teaspoons milk (use casein-free vanilla soy or
    rice milk for dairy-free diets)
1 teaspoon vanilla
1 tablespoon + 2 teaspoons vegetable oil
1 tablespoon + 1 teaspoon grated dark chocolate

1. In a medium bowl, whisk together the flour mixture, sugar, baking powder, salt, and cocoa.
2. Break the egg into the flour mixture, and then add the milk, vanilla, and oil.
3. Use a wire whisk to thoroughly mix all the ingredients.
4. Stir in the grated chocolate.
5. Spray a large, 1½-cup mug or 1½-cup glass bowl with nonstick spray.
6. With a rubber spatula, scrape the batter into the mug or bowl.
7. Put it in the microwave for 3 minutes on high power.
8. When it's done cooking, tip the cake onto a dish, cut it in half, and enjoy!

*Makes 2 (¾-cup) servings*

One serving—Calories: 413; Total fat: 18.3 g; Saturated fat: 4 g; Cholesterol: 108 mg; Sodium: 90 mg; Carbohydrates: 59.9 g; Fiber: 2.6 g; Sugar: 39.3 g; Protein: 5.3 g

## Molasses Cake

1 cup milk (use casein-free vanilla soy or rice milk for dairy-free diets)

1 teaspoon cider vinegar

1 egg

1 teaspoon vanilla

¼ cup + 2 tablespoons vegetable oil

2¼ cups sugar

2 teaspoons baking soda

1 teaspoon cinnamon

¼ teaspoon ground cloves

¼ teaspoon ground ginger

¼ teaspoon salt

1¾ cups gluten-free flour mixture (See the Gluten-Free Flour Mixtures on page 16)

½ cup molasses

½ cup raisins

1. Preheat the oven to 350°F. Spray a 9-inch square baking pan with nonstick spray.
2. Pour the milk into a small bowl. Add the vinegar, then set the bowl aside. The milk will soon start to look like it is curdling.
3. In a large bowl, whisk the egg. Add the vanilla, oil, and sugar and whisk till blended.
4. Add the milk mixture and whisk again to blend.
5. Add the baking soda, cinnamon, cloves, ginger, salt, and flour mixture. Use a rubber spatula to mix ingredients.
6. Add the molasses and raisins and stir to blend well.
7. Pour batter into the baking pan and bake for 40 to 45 minutes or until a toothpick inserted in the center comes out clean.

**Note:** Molasses is very sticky. The easiest way to measure it is to spray the measuring cup with nonstick spray before pouring in the molasses. With the spray, the sticky molasses will slide right out!

*Makes 12 (3″ × 2¼″) servings*

One serving—Calories: 356; Total fat: 8.4 g; Saturated fat: 1.1 g; Cholesterol: 9 mg; Sodium: 279 mg; Carbohydrates: 72.1 g; Fiber: 1.2 g; Sugar: 50 g; Protein: 2 g

## Almond Cake

**Cake**

> 2 eggs
> ⅔ cup butter, melted and slightly cooled (use dairy-free margarine for dairy-free diets)
> ½ cup granulated sugar
> ½ teaspoon almond flavoring
> 1½ teaspoons vanilla
> 1 cup gluten-free flour mixture (See the Gluten-Free Flour Mixtures on page 16)
> 2 teaspoons baking powder

## Topping

> ½ cup brown sugar
>
> 3 tablespoons butter (use dairy-free margarine for dairy-free diets)
>
> 2 tablespoons milk (use casein-free soy, rice, or almond milk for dairy-free diets)
>
> ⅓ cup finely chopped almonds

1. Preheat oven to 350°F. Spray a 9-inch square baking pan with nonstick spray.
2. In a large bowl, whisk the eggs until they are frothy.
3. Add the melted butter and stir well. Then add the granulated sugar, almond flavoring, and vanilla and whisk to blend ingredients.
4. With a rubber spatula, stir in the flour mixture and baking powder. When all of the ingredients are well blended together, spoon the batter into the baking pan.
5. Bake for 20 minutes or until light golden and toothpick inserted in center comes out clean.
6. Remove cake from the oven and prick it all over with a wooden skewer. Poke the holes all the way to the bottom of the cake because you want the topping to partially seep through the cake.
7. Set the oven to broil.
8. Put the brown sugar, butter, and milk in a small saucepan. Stir with a wooden spoon, over medium heat, until the butter melts and the mixture is smooth. Remove the pan from the heat and stir in the almonds. Pour this mixture over the hot cake, smoothing out the top with the back of a spoon.
9. Put the cake in the oven and broil for 2 to 3 minutes or until the topping is caramelized and golden. (Check the cake every 15 seconds to make sure the almonds don't burn.)
10. Leave the cake in the baking pan to cool and so the sauce can soak through the cake.

**Note:** The quickest way to melt butter for the cake is to place the butter in a glass measuring cup, cover it well with wax paper, and then microwave it for 40 seconds or until the butter has completely melted. If you prefer a frosted cake, eliminate the topping above and frost the cooled cake with your favorite icing.

*Makes 12 (3" × 2¼") servings*

One serving with topping—Calories: 252; Total fat: 15.3 g; Saturated fat: 8.6 g; Cholesterol: 70 mg; Sodium: 168 mg; Carbohydrates: 31.8 g; Fiber: 0.8 g; Sugar: 17.6 g; Protein: 2.2 g

## Apple Cake

2 eggs

½ cup vegetable oil

¼ cup water

1 teaspoon vanilla

½ teaspoon salt

1 cup gluten-free flour mixture
    (See the Gluten-Free Flour
    Mixtures on page 16)

2 teaspoons baking soda

1 cup granulated sugar

1 teaspoon cinnamon

1 (21-ounce) can apple pie filling

1 cup chopped walnuts

¼ cup powdered sugar

1 Preheat oven to 350°F. Spray an 8" × 12" baking pan with nonstick spray.

2 Whisk the eggs in a large bowl until very frothy. Whisk in the oil, water, and vanilla.

3 Add the salt, flour mixture, baking soda, granulated sugar, and cinnamon, and then stir with a rubber spatula until completely combined.

④ Empty the pie filling into a small bowl. Cut the apples in it into small pieces. Stir the pie filling and walnuts into the batter.

⑤ Pour the batter into the pan. Bake for 40 minutes or until a toothpick inserted in the center comes out clean.

⑥ Once the cake has cooled, sift powdered sugar over the top of the cake.

*Makes 12 (4″ × 2″) servings*

One serving—Calories: 299; Total fat: 16.7 g; Saturated fat: 1.6 g; Cholesterol: 35 mg; Sodium: 342 mg; Carbohydrates: 42.4 g; Fiber: 1.7 g; Sugar: 25.9 g; Protein: 3 g

## Chocolate Cherry Cake

2 eggs
¾ cup vegetable oil
1 tablespoon vanilla
¾ cup sugar
1 teaspoon cinnamon
1 tablespoon baking soda
1 teaspoon baking powder
2 cups gluten-free flour mixture (See the Gluten-Free Flour
    Mixtures on page 16)
1 (21-ounce) can cherry pie filling
¾ cup chopped dark chocolate

① Preheat oven to 350°F. Spray an 8½″ × 11″ baking pan with nonstick spray.

② In a medium bowl, whisk the eggs until frothy. Whip in the oil, vanilla, sugar, and cinnamon.

③ Add the baking soda, baking powder, and flour mixture and stir with a rubber spatula until blended.

④ Fold in the cherry pie filling and chocolate.

⑤ Spoon the batter into the baking pan. Bake for 40 minutes or until a toothpick inserted in the center comes out clean.

*Makes 12 (2¾" × 2¾") servings*

One serving—Calories: 442; Total fat: 15.6 g; Saturated fat: 4.2 g; Cholesterol: 2 mg; Sodium: 326 mg; Carbohydrates: 70.3 g; Fiber: 3.1 g; Sugar: 18.7 g; Protein: 2.3 g

## Mississippi Mud Cake

5 eggs

3 tablespoons milk (use casein-free vanilla soy
    or rice milk for dairy-free diets)

2 teaspoons vanilla

2 cups granulated sugar

⅓ cup unsweetened cocoa

1⅔ cups gluten-free flour mixture
    (See the Gluten-Free Flour
    Mixtures on page 16)

1 tablespoon baking powder

1 cup chopped walnuts

¾ cup finely chopped dark chocolate

2 jars (7 ounces each) marshmallow cream (Suzanne's Ricemellow
    Crème is gluten- and dairy-free)

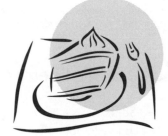

**Frosting**

½ cup butter (use dairy-free margarine for dairy-free diets)

⅓ cup unsweetened cocoa

2 cups sifted powdered sugar

⅓ cup milk (use casein-free soy or rice milk for dairy-free diets)

1 teaspoon vanilla

1. Preheat oven to 350°F. Spray a 9" × 13" baking pan with non-stick spray.

2. In a medium bowl, whisk the eggs, milk, and vanilla until frothy. Add the granulated sugar and whisk again.

3. Sift the cocoa, flour mixture, and baking powder into a small bowl, and then stir into the egg mixture. Stir in the walnuts and chocolate pieces.

4. Spoon the batter into the baking pan. Smooth the top of the batter with a wet rubber spatula.

5. Bake for 25 minutes or until a toothpick inserted in the center comes out clean.

6. While the cake is still hot, put spoonfuls of the marshmallow cream on top of the cake. Let it set for 2 to 3 minutes to soften, and then spread it over the top of the cake with the back of a wet spoon. Let cake cool for 10 minutes before spreading the chocolate frosting.

7. To make the frosting, melt the butter in a medium saucepan. When melted, remove the pan from the stove.

8. Sift the cocoa and powdered sugar onto a piece of wax paper. Carefully lift the wax paper, and pour the cocoa and sugar mixture into the saucepan with the melted margarine. Stir until blended. Stir in the milk and vanilla.

9. Spread the icing over the slightly warm cake. (If the frosting is too thick to spread, add a little more milk.)

*Makes 24 (3" × 1½") servings*

One serving—Calories: 267; Total fat: 8.7 g; Saturated fat: 3.9 g; Cholesterol: 55 mg; Sodium: 103 mg; Carbohydrates: 87.5 g; Fiber: 1.4 g; Sugar: 55.7 g; Protein: 5.4 g

## Upside-Down Fruit Salad Cake

1½ cups gluten-free flour mixture (See the Gluten-Free Flour Mixtures on page 16)

2 teaspoons baking soda

1½ teaspoons baking powder

½ teaspoon salt

¾ teaspoon cinnamon

¼ teaspoon nutmeg

1 cup sugar

⅔ cup vegetable oil

¼ cup orange juice

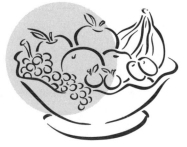

2 eggs

2 teaspoons vanilla

½ cup blueberries, washed and drained

1 large banana, diced

¼ cup shredded coconut

1 (8-ounce) can crushed pineapple, undrained

½ cup chopped pecans

1. Preheat oven to 350°F. Spray an 8″ × 12″ baking pan with nonstick spray.
2. In a medium bowl, whisk together the flour mixture, baking soda, baking powder, salt, cinnamon, and nutmeg.
3. In a large bowl, whisk together the sugar, oil, juice, eggs, and vanilla until smooth. Using a rubber spatula, stir the flour mixture into the large bowl, mixing until the ingredients are combined.
4. Gently fold in the blueberries, banana, coconut, pineapple, and pecans.
5. Pour the batter into the pan. Bake for 50 minutes or until a toothpick inserted in the center comes out clean.
6. Cool the pan on a wire rack.

*Makes 12 (4″ × 2″) servings*

One serving—Calories: 314; Total fat: 17.2 g; Saturated fat: 2 g; Cholesterol: 35 mg; Sodium: 370 mg; Carbohydrates: 39.1 g; Fiber: 2 g; Sugar: 22.4 g; Protein: 2.4 g

## Fruited Pears

1 pear, cut in half lengthwise and cored

8 pitted dates, chopped

32 raisins

3 tablespoons chopped walnuts

2 tablespoons pineapple preserves

1. Set the pear halves in a small microwave-safe baking dish. Add enough water around the pears so the water is about 1 inch deep (about ½ cup).
2. In a small bowl, stir together the dates, raisins, walnuts, and preserves until combined. Spoon this mixture over the tops of the pear halves.
3. Microwave on high for 5 minutes or until the pears are fork-tender.

**Note:** If you chop dates with a knife, they get very sticky. The easiest way to "chop" dates is to cut them into small pieces with a pair of clean scissors.

*Makes 2 servings*

One serving—Calories: 469; Total fat: 7.4 g; Saturated fat: 0.7 g; Cholesterol: 0 mg; Sodium: 9 mg; Carbohydrates: 107.6 g; Fiber: 10.4 g; Sugar: 90 g; Protein: 4.1 g

## 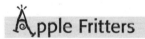 Apple Fritters

1 egg

⅔ cup granulated sugar

1 cup milk (use casein-free soy or rice milk for dairy-free diets)

3 tablespoons orange juice

1 tablespoon vanilla

2 teaspoons cinnamon

¼ teaspoon nutmeg

¼ teaspoon salt

1 tablespoon baking powder

2 teaspoons baking soda

2 cups gluten-free flour mixture (See the Gluten-Free Flour Mixtures on page 16)

1 medium apple, peeled, cored, and chopped fine

2 cups vegetable oil

Sifted powdered sugar

1. In a large bowl, whisk the egg until light and fluffy. Add the granulated sugar, milk, orange juice, and vanilla and whisk until blended.

2. Add the cinnamon, nutmeg, salt, baking powder, baking soda, and flour mixture; mix well with a rubber spatula.

3. Stir in the apple pieces. Let batter rest for 3 minutes to thicken.

4. Line a colander with several sheets of paper toweling; set aside.

5. Heat the oil in a small saucepan for 1 minute over medium heat. Working in small batches, drop fritter batter by tea-spoonfuls into the oil. Fry until fritters are golden brown on all sides (2 to 3 minutes). Remove the fritters from the oil with a fork or slotted spoon and drain them in the colander.

6. When fritters have cooled, dust tops with sifted powdered sugar.

**Note:** Hot oil can burn the skin badly. Children should definitely have adult supervision when frying the fritters.

*Makes 40 fritters*

One fritter—Calories: 52; Total fat: 1.1 g; Saturated fat: 0.2 g; Cholesterol: 6 mg; Sodium: 109 mg; Carbohydrates: 10.6 g; Fiber: 0.4 g; Sugar: 4.1 g; Protein: 0.6 g

## Berry Crisp

    5 cups fresh strawberries
    2 cups fresh blueberries (2 packages, 4.4 ounces each)
    ½ cup coarsely chopped pecans
    ⅔ cup sugar
    5 teaspoons cornstarch
    3 tablespoons orange juice
    1 cup crushed gluten-free shortbread cookies (about 12 small
        cookies) (Shortcake Rings from Glutano are gluten- and
        dairy-free)

1. Preheat the oven to 375°F. Spray a 9-inch pie plate with non-stick spray.
2. Wash and drain the strawberries and blueberries.
3. Cut the tops off the strawberries, then cut each strawberry into 8 pieces.
4. Put the blueberries and strawberries into a large bowl. Add the pecans, sugar, and cornstarch and stir to blend. Spoon the berry mixture into the pie plate.
5. Drizzle the orange juice over the berries.
6. Sprinkle the cookie crumbs over the fruit.
7. Bake for 30 minutes or until the filling is bubbling and the crumbs on top are slightly golden.

**Note:** The following calorie count is based on using vanilla shortbread cookies, but other cookies you can use include cinnamon, lemon, or gingerbread cookies.

*Makes 8 servings*

One serving—Calories: 226; Total fat: 7.1 g; Saturated fat: 1.2 g; Cholesterol: 0 mg; Sodium: 23 mg; Carbohydrates: 41.5 g; Fiber: 3.4 g; Sugar: 26.94 g; Protein: 2.2 g

# Frozen Chocolate Peanut Butter Pie

**Crust**

1 cup peanut butter

1 cup corn syrup

4 cups gluten-free puffed rice cereal (Earth's Best makes gluten- and dairy-free puffed rice cereal)

**Filling**

1 pint chocolate ice cream, partially softened (Turtle Mountain makes gluten- and dairy-free ice cream)

¾ cup peanut butter

### Frosting

4 tablespoons butter (use stick dairy-free margarine for dairy-free diets)

⅓ cup unsweetened cocoa

½ teaspoon vanilla

1½ cups sifted powdered sugar

2 tablespoons milk (use casein-free vanilla soy or rice milk for dairy-free diets)

2 tablespoons chopped peanuts

1. To make the crust, use a rubber spatula to blend the peanut butter and corn syrup in a medium bowl. Add the cereal, and mix well. Press the mixture into a 9-inch pie plate that has been sprayed with nonstick spray.

2. To make the filling, spoon the ice cream into a bowl. With a whisk, fold in the peanut butter so it is streaked through the ice cream. Spoon the filling into the piecrust.

3. To make the frosting, melt the butter in a medium saucepan. Remove the pan from the stove. Stir in the cocoa and vanilla. Whisk in half of the powdered sugar, then half of the milk till blended, then whisk in the remaining powdered sugar and the remaining milk. Beat with a whisk until the frosting is just thin enough to spread. (Add 1 tablespoon more milk if needed.) Using a knife, spread the frosting on the pie. Sprinkle peanuts on top of the frosting.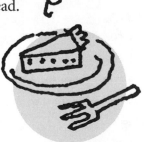

4. Cover the pie with foil. Freeze until firm, about 4 hours.

*Makes 8 servings*

One serving—Calories: 690; Total fat: 38 g; Saturated fat: 11.1 g; Cholesterol: 21 mg; Sodium: 219 mg; Carbohydrates: 81.8 g; Fiber: 5.1 g; Sugar: 41.6 g; Protein: 17.2 g

# Cheesecake Pie

## Crust

1⅓ cups finely crushed gluten-free crisp cookies (Glutano
    Shortcake Rings or Josef's Sugar Cookies are gluten- and
    dairy-free)

¼ teaspoon cinnamon

¼ cup butter, softened (use dairy-free margarine for dairy-free
    diets)

## Filling

1 (8-ounce) package cream cheese, at room temperature (Vegan
    Gourmet Cream Cheese Alternative is gluten- and dairy-free)

2 eggs

1 teaspoon vanilla

½ teaspoon almond or lemon flavoring

½ cup sugar

1. Preheat oven to 350°F. Lightly spray a 9-inch pie plate with nonstick spray.

2. Put the cookie crumbs, cinnamon, and butter in a medium bowl. With a fork, mix the ingredients well. Press the mixture onto the bottom and sides of the pie plate. Set crust aside.

3. Put the cream cheese, eggs, vanilla, flavoring, and sugar into a blender. Puree for 20 seconds. Remove lid and scrape down sides of blender. Cover blender and puree for 20 more seconds or until ingredients are smooth and thoroughly combined.

4. Pour the cream cheese mixture into the piecrust. Bake for 25 minutes or until the center is just set. Do not refrigerate the cheesecake until it has cooled completely.

*Makes 8 servings*

One serving—Calories: 246; Total fat: 18.1 g; Saturated fat: 9.9 g; Cholesterol: 100 mg; Sodium: 177 mg; Carbohydrates: 17.7 g; Fiber: 0.1 g; Sugar: 14.5 g; Protein: 3.7 g

# Chocolate Chip Pie

3 eggs

1½ teaspoons vanilla

⅔ cup vegetable oil

½ cup granulated sugar

½ cup brown sugar

⅔ cup gluten-free flour mixture (See the Gluten-Free Flour Mixtures
   on page 16)

2 teaspoons baking powder

¾ cup chopped dark chocolate

1 cup chopped walnuts

1 Preheat oven to 325°F. Spray a 10-inch pie plate with nonstick spray.

2 In a large bowl, whip the eggs and vanilla with a whisk until foamy. Add the oil and blend together. Whisk in the granulated sugar and brown sugar.

3 With a rubber spatula, stir in the flour mixture and baking powder. Stir well until all ingredients are blended.

4 Stir in the chocolate chips and walnuts.

5 Pour the batter into the pie plate.

6 Bake for 50 minutes or until a toothpick inserted in the center comes out clean.

*Makes 8 servings*

One serving—Calories: 537; Total fat: 37.2 g; Saturated fat: 7.2 g; Cholesterol: 82 mg; Sodium: 131 mg; Carbohydrates: 51.3 g; Fiber: 3.2 g; Sugar: 37.9 g; Protein: 3.2 g

# Apple Cranberry Cobbler

1 (21-ounce) can apple pie filling

1 (16-ounce) can whole-berry cranberry sauce

¼ cup gluten-free flour mixture (See the Gluten-Free Flour Mixtures
   on page 16)

½ teaspoon cinnamon

¼ cup brown sugar

½ cup chopped walnuts

⅓ cup butter (use dairy-free margarine for dairy-free diets)

1. Preheat oven to 400°F. Spray a 9-inch square baking pan with nonstick spray.
2. In a medium bowl, stir together the pie filling and cranberry sauce. Spoon mixture into the baking pan.
3. In a small bowl, stir together the flour mixture, cinnamon, brown sugar, and nuts. Sprinkle this mixture over the apple-cranberry filling.
4. Put butter in a glass measuring cup and heat in the microwave on high for 50 seconds or until it is melted. Slowly pour this over the top of the dessert.
5. Bake for 25 minutes or until the whole dessert is bubbling. May be served warm or at room temperature.

*Makes 8 servings*

One serving—Calories: 376; Total fat: 20.1 g; Saturated fat: 10.2 g; Cholesterol: 40 mg; Sodium: 160 mg; Carbohydrates: 50.8 g; Fiber: 3 g; Sugar: 36.8 g; Protein: 2.4 g

## Peach Bread Pudding

3 eggs

¾ cup brown sugar

¼ teaspoon salt

1 cup milk

1½ teaspoons vanilla

½ teaspoon nutmeg

1 teaspoon cinnamon

4 slices gluten-free bread, cut into small cubes

½ cup raisins

1 (8¾-ounce) can peaches, drained and diced

1. Preheat oven to 350°F. Spray an 8-inch square baking pan with nonstick spray.
2. In a large bowl, whip the eggs with a whisk until frothy.
3. Add the brown sugar, salt, milk, vanilla, nutmeg, and cinnamon. Whisk until the ingredients are blended.
4. Stir in the bread cubes, raisins, and peaches. (In place of peaches, you can use blueberries.)
5. Pour the pudding into the pan. Let the pan set on the counter for 30 minutes so the bread can absorb some of the liquid, then bake for 40 minutes.

*Makes 9 (2⅔-inch square) servings*

One serving—Calories: 179; Total fat: 3.2 g; Saturated fat: 1.1 g; Cholesterol: 73 mg; Sodium: 158 mg; Carbohydrates: 43.4 g; Fiber: 1.4 g; Sugar: 27.7 g; Protein: 4.4 g

## Butterscotch Pudding

3 eggs

1 teaspoon vanilla

1½ cups milk (use casein-free vanilla soy or rice milk for dairy-free diets)

1 cup brown sugar

2 tablespoons cornstarch

¼ teaspoon salt

2 tablespoons butter, melted and cooled (use dairy-free margarine for dairy-free diets)

1. In a medium bowl, whisk the eggs until very frothy. Whisk in the vanilla and milk.
2. Add the brown sugar, cornstarch, and salt and whisk until completely blended and mixture is smooth.
3. Whisk in the melted butter.
4. Pour pudding into an 8-inch square microwave-safe baking dish that has been sprayed with nonstick spray. Microwave on

high for 4 to 6 minutes, stirring mixture every 1½ minutes, until pudding has thickened.

*Makes 9 servings*

One serving—Calories: 172; Total fat: 5.5 g; Saturated fat: 2.9 g; Cholesterol: 81 mg; Sodium: 134 mg; Carbohydrates: 36.5 g; Fiber: 0.01 g; Sugar: 26 g; Protein: 3.5 g

# Fruity French Toast Wraps

1 egg

½ cup milk (use casein-free vanilla soy milk or almond milk for dairy-free diets)

¼ teaspoon vanilla

¼ teaspoon cinnamon

½ teaspoon sugar

2 gluten-free flour tortillas

½ cup canned pie filling

1. In a pie plate, use a wire whisk to mix together the egg, milk, vanilla, cinnamon, and sugar.
2. Spray a large nonstick skillet with nonstick spray. Heat the skillet over medium-high heat until it is hot.
3. Place one tortilla in the egg mixture, turning it to coat it on both sides.
4. Cook the tortilla in the hot skillet, about 2 minutes per side, until golden. Remove it from the pan and place it on a dish. Repeat this procedure with the second tortilla. (Be careful how you handle the tortillas because they will be very hot when they come out of the skillet.)
5. Spoon ¼ cup pie filling along one side of each tortilla, then tightly roll up the tortilla.

*Makes 2 (1-tortilla) servings*

One serving—Calories: 275; Total fat: 7.6 g; Saturated fat: 2.3 g; Cholesterol: 112 mg; Sodium: 331 mg; Carbohydrates: 42.3 g; Fiber: 0.6 g; Sugar: 11.3 g; Protein: 9.6 g

## Peanut Butter Baked Apples

This recipe is also good using pears instead of apples.

  2 apples, any variety
  4 tablespoons peanut butter
  2 teaspoons finely chopped dark chocolate

1 Preheat oven to 350°F. Spray an 8-inch square baking pan with nonstick spray.

2 Cut each apple in half lengthwise and core (cut out the seeds).

3 Spread one side of each apple half with 1 tablespoon of the peanut butter. Place the apple halves in the baking pan, peanut butter-side up.

4 Sprinkle the chocolate on top of the peanut butter.

5 Bake the apples for about 15 minutes or until the chocolate has melted. Caution: apples will be very hot. Let them cool before eating them.

*Makes 4 (½-apple) servings*

One serving—Calories: 153; Total fat: 9 g; Saturated fat: 2.1 g; Cholesterol: 0 mg; Sodium: 5 mg; Carbohydrates: 17.2 g; Fiber: 3.3 g; Sugar: 2.4 g; Protein: 4.4 g

## Winter Fruit Bowl

  1 (15-ounce) can fruit cocktail
  1 (10-ounce) package frozen strawberries, thawed but not drained
  1 cup frozen blueberries, thawed
  1 banana
  ½ cup mini marshmallows (AllerEnergy makes dairy-free
      marshmallows)
  ½ cup shredded coconut

1 Pour the fruit cocktail into a strainer to drain off the juice. Put the drained fruit in a medium bowl.

2 Add the strawberries (with their juice) to the bowl.

③ Stir in the blueberries.

④ Peel the banana. Slice the banana into the fruit bowl.

⑤ Stir in the marshmallows and coconut.

⑥ Cover the bowl with plastic wrap. Refrigerate fruit for 1 hour to blend flavors.

*Makes 6 (1-cup) servings*

One serving—Calories: 118; Total fat: 2.3 g; Saturated fat: 1.9 g; Cholesterol: 0 mg; Sodium: 27 mg; Carbohydrates: 25.7 g; Fiber: 3.5 g; Sugar: 17.9 g; Protein: 1 g

## Apple and Pear Dip

1 (8-ounce) package cream cheese,
    softened (Vegan Gourmet
    makes gluten- and dairy-free
    cream cheese alternative)
1 cup finely chopped dark chocolate
½ cup chopped walnuts
Apples and pears for dipping

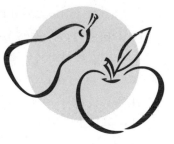

① Spread the cream cheese on the bottom of a 9-inch glass pie plate. Sprinkle the chocolate over the cheese. Sprinkle the nuts over the chocolate.

② Microwave on medium (50 percent power) for 3 to 4 minutes or until warm.

③ Slice and core the apples and pears for dipping into the sauce.

**Note:** You can add coconut or spread creamy peanut butter on top of the cream cheese before sprinkling the chocolate. You can also use chopped peanuts in place of the walnuts.

*Makes 8 (¼-cup) servings*

One serving (dip only)—Calories: 289; Total fat: 24.1 g; Saturated fat: 11.5 g; Cholesterol: 35 mg; Sodium: 103 mg; Carbohydrates: 20.6 g; Fiber: 2.9 g; Sugar: 16.3 g; Protein: 4.4 g

# Flowerpot Sundaes

6 gluten-free chocolate cookies, crushed (Enjoy Life chocolate
cookies, Curious Cookie's chocolate cookies, and Nana's
Chocolate Crunch Cookies are gluten- and dairy-free)

1 quart of your favorite flavor of ice cream (Turtle Mountain makes
dairy-free ice cream)

¼ cup shredded coconut

Few drops green food coloring

**You'll Need**

6 (8-ounce) Styrofoam cups

6 plastic flowers

1 Set aside half of the crushed cookies. Spoon the remaining
half of the cookies into the bottoms of 6 Styrofoam cups,
dividing evenly.

2 Add a scoop of ice cream to cover the cookies in each cup.

3 Sprinkle the reserved cookie crumbs equally on top of the ice
cream to look like soil.

4 Place the coconut in a sandwich-size, self-seal plastic bag. Add
a few drops of green food coloring. Seal the bag, and mix well
to distribute the coloring evenly. Sprinkle the coconut on top
of the sundaes.

5 Place a plastic flower in each cup.

6 Freeze the cups for a minimum of 3 hours before serving.

*Makes 6 sundaes*

One sundae—Calories: 258; Total fat: 12.9 g; Saturated fat: 7.4 g; Cholesterol: 39 mg;
Sodium: 133 mg; Carbohydrates: 26 g; Fiber: 2 g; Sugar: 26 g; Protein: 3.7 g

# Hot Banana Sundae

1 banana, unpeeled

1 teaspoon honey

1 teaspoon brown sugar

¼ teaspoon cinnamon

1 scoop (½ cup) vanilla ice cream
(Turtle Mountain makes dairy-free
ice cream)

1 Preheat oven to 350°F.

2 Split the unpeeled banana lengthwise.

3 Drizzle half of the honey on each banana half.

4 Sprinkle each half with the brown sugar and cinnamon.

5 Put the halves of the banana back together. Wrap the banana in two layers of foil. Place the foil packet directly on a rack in the middle of the oven. Bake for 10 minutes.

6 Put the ice cream into a small bowl. Carefully scoop out the baked banana, and spoon it over the ice cream. (The banana will be hot, so be careful not to burn yourself.)

*Makes 1 sundae*

One sundae—Calories: 282; Total fat: 7.7 g; Saturated fat: 4.6 g; Cholesterol: 29 mg; Sodium: 55 mg; Carbohydrates: 53.3 g; Fiber: 3.9 g; Sugar: 38.6 g; Protein: 3.7 g

# Fruity Pops

½ cup crushed pineapple

½ cup frozen strawberries, thawed

2 cups vanilla ice cream, softened (Turtle Mountain makes dairy-free ice cream)

1 (12-ounce) can frozen orange-pineapple juice concentrate, thawed

**You'll Need**

8 (5-ounce) paper cups

8 wooden Popsicle sticks

1. Drain the pineapple and strawberries in a strainer. Discard juices.
2. Put the pineapple, strawberries, ice cream, and juice concentrate into a medium-size bowl. Mix them together till completely blended.
3. Spoon the mixture into the paper cups. Stretch a piece of plastic wrap across the top of each cup.
4. Using a Popsicle stick, poke a hole in the plastic wrap. Stand the stick straight up in the center of the cup.
5. Freeze the cups for 4 or more hours.
6. Remove the plastic wrap, and peel away each paper cup before serving.

*Makes 8 fruity pops*

One fruity pop—Calories: 165; Total fat: 3.8 g; Saturated fat: 2.3 g; Cholesterol: 14 mg; Sodium: 28 mg; Carbohydrates: 31.3 g; Fiber: 1.1 g; Sugar: 29.3 g; Protein: 2.5 g

## Peanut Butter Pops

   1 envelope unflavored gelatin
   3 tablespoons grated dark chocolate
   1 cup boiling water
   1 cup peanut butter
   1 cup milk (use casein-free soy milk or almond milk for dairy-free
      diets)

**You'll Need**

   10 (5-ounce) paper cups
   10 Popsicle sticks

1. In a medium bowl, mix the gelatin and grated chocolate with the boiling water, stirring until the gelatin is completely dissolved.
2. With a whisk, blend in the peanut butter.
3. Stir in the milk.

4 Pour the mixture into the paper cups. Freeze the cups for 45 minutes until mixture begins to thicken, then insert a Popsicle stick into the center of each cup.

5 Freeze pops for 4 hours or until firm.

*Makes 10 peanut butter pops*

One peanut butter pop—Calories: 190; Total fat: 15.2 g; Saturated fat: 5.5 g; Cholesterol: 3 mg; Sodium: 17 mg; Carbohydrates: 8.9 g; Fiber: 1.9 g; Sugar: 5.9 g; Protein: 8.1 g

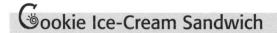

## Cookie Ice-Cream Sandwich

2 gluten-free cookies (Pamela's has gluten- and dairy-free cookies)

¼ cup ice cream (your favorite flavor) or sherbet (Turtle Mountain makes dairy-free ice cream)

Chopped nuts, multicolored sprinkles, coconut, or grated dark chocolate

1 Put one cookie on a dish, top down.

2 Put the scoop of ice cream on top of the cookie.

3 Place the remaining cookie on top of the ice cream or sherbet, top up. Roll the edges in the nuts, sprinkles, coconut, and/or grated chocolate.

4 Wrap the ice-cream sandwich in foil. Freeze for 4 hours or until firm.

### Sandwich Suggestions

Chocolate chip cookies (made with dark chocolate for dairy-free diets) with vanilla ice cream rolled in shaved dark chocolate

Peanut butter cookies with chocolate ice cream rolled in chopped peanuts

Sugar cookies with peach ice cream rolled in chopped walnuts

Lemon cookies with lemon sherbet rolled in coconut

Orange cookies with orange sorbet rolled in multicolored sprinkles

*Makes 1 ice-cream sandwich*

One ice-cream sandwich (chocolate chip cookie, vanilla ice cream, and 1 tablespoon chopped walnuts)—Calories: 205; Total fat: 11.3 g; Saturated fat: 3.4 g; Cholesterol: 15 mg; Sodium: 101 mg; Carbohydrates: 23.4 g; Fiber: 1.4 g; Sugar: 7.2 g; Protein: 3.4 g

# Crunchy Ice-Cream Sandwiches

3 cups gluten-free puffed rice cereal (Erewhon Crispy Brown Rice
    Cereal is gluten- and dairy-free)
½ cup minced dark chocolate
1½ cups peanut butter
1 pint of your favorite flavor of ice cream, slightly softened (Turtle
    Mountain makes dairy-free ice cream)

1 In a large bowl, mix the cereal, dark chocolate, and peanut butter until well blended. Spread half of the mixture in an 9-inch square pan.

2 Carefully spread the ice cream over the cereal layer.

3 Spread the remaining cereal mixture on top of the ice cream, smoothing out the top.

4 Cover the pan with foil. Freeze for 3 hours. Cut into 3-inch squares to serve.

*Makes 9 servings*

One serving—Calories: 414; Total fat: 29.2 g; Saturated fat: 8.9 g; Cholesterol: 14 mg; Sodium: 121 mg; Carbohydrates: 31.5 g; Fiber: 3.9 g; Sugar: 17.8 g; Protein: 13.2 g

# Personalized Parfaits

1 pint vanilla ice cream (Turtle Mountain makes dairy-free ice
    cream)
1 pint chocolate ice cream

**Toppings**

Crushed gluten-free cookies (Gluten-Free Pantry has gluten- and dairy-free chocolate chip cookies)

Finely chopped dark chocolate

Mini marshmallows (AllerEnergy makes dairy-free marshmallows)

Chopped nuts

Pineapple preserves

Maraschino cherries

Strawberry pie filling

Multicolored sprinkles

1 Using an ice-cream scoop, scoop the ice creams into balls and place on a cookie sheet. (Work quickly so the ice cream doesn't start to melt.) Freeze the ice-cream balls until ready to serve.

2 Set out eight small bowls. Spoon a different topping into each of the bowls.

3 When ready to serve, transfer the ice-cream balls to a medium bowl.

4 Give everyone a parfait glass or dessert bowl. Place the bowls of toppings in the center of the table, and let everyone make a parfait.

*Makes 8 parfaits*

One parfait (1 scoop vanilla ice cream, 2 tablespoons strawberry pie filling, and 2 teaspoons multicolored sprinkles)—Calories: 160; Total fat: 7.9 g; Saturated fat: 4.5 g; Cholesterol: 29 mg; Sodium: 55 mg; Carbohydrates: 19.9 g; Fiber: 5.2 g; Sugar: 17.9 g; Protein: 2.3 g

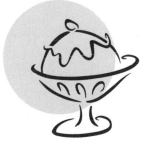

# 8

# Kitchen Projects

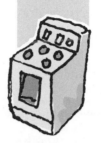

## Pomander Ball

Place the pomander on the kitchen counter to make the kitchen smell good. Or make several pomanders, and arrange them in a bowl for a sweet-smelling centerpiece.

Thin ribbon
1 small orange, unpeeled
½ teaspoon cinnamon
100 whole cloves

1. Tie the ribbon around the orange, making a bow at the top.
2. Put the cinnamon in a sandwich-size, reclosable plastic bag. Add the cloves. Seal the bag, and shake it to coat the cloves with the cinnamon.
3. Push the cloves into the orange. Continue inserting cloves until the entire surface of the orange is covered (except where the ribbon is).

**Note:** If the skin of the orange is too thick, the stems of the cloves may break off when you try to insert them. To avoid this, prick the orange with the tip of a skewer before inserting the clove.

## Homemade Play Dough

Store in a self-seal bag to keep the dough pliable.

½ cup peanut butter

¼ cup honey

1 cup cornmeal

2 teaspoons cream of tartar

1 In a medium bowl, stir together the peanut butter and honey.

2 With your hands, work in the cornmeal and cream of tartar until completely blended.

3 Store the dough in a self-seal bag.

**Note:** It may be necessary to add a little bit more cornmeal or a little bit more peanut butter to get the right consistency. Do not refrigerate the dough or it will become too hard.

## Kitchen Garden

As the days pass, you will see your vegetable or pineapple grow roots. Organic vegetables and fruits sprout sooner and healthier because they are not treated with growth retardants and inhibitors.

1 widemouthed glass jar or plastic bowl

4 to 6 toothpicks

1 organic potato, sweet potato, yam, or pineapple top

1. Fill the jar or bowl with water.
2. Push toothpicks into the vegetable or fruit so that the toothpicks balance on the outside rim of the container and the bottom part of the fruit is partially immersed in the water.
3. Set the container on the kitchen counter for several weeks. Add water every few days to keep the bottom part of the vegetable or fruit in water.

## Bubbles

You can create these fun bubbles using a slotted spoon if you don't have an empty spool.

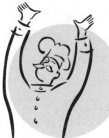

2 cups warm water
2 tablespoons liquid dish detergent
1 tablespoon sugar
1 empty thread spool

1. In a bowl, stir together the water, detergent, and sugar.
2. Dip one end of the spool into the soap mixture. Blow bubbles through the spool from the dry end.

## Tree Ornaments

The variety of ornaments you can make is unlimited.

2 cups gluten-free flour mixture (See the Gluten-Free Flour
    Mixtures on page 16)
1 cup salt
¾ to 1 cup water
Cookie cutters (optional)
Paints (water, acrylic, or oil-based)
Clear varnish
String

1. Preheat oven to 325°F.
2. Stir the flour mixture and salt together in a medium bowl.
3. Add ¾ cup of water and stir. If the mixture is too dry, add another ¼ cup of water.
4. Knead the dough for 5 minutes.
5. With a rolling pin, roll out the dough on a cutting board to ¼ inch thick.
6. Use large cookie cutters to cut out shapes.
7. Use a straw or similarly sized implement to make a hole near the top of each shape for hanging the ornament.
8. Line a cookie sheet with foil.
9. Place the ornaments on top of the foil.
10. Bake for 35 to 40 minutes or until the ornaments are hard.
11. Remove the hot tray from the oven. Let the ornaments cool completely.
12. Paint the ornaments. Once the paint has thoroughly dried, apply a coat of varnish to all sides to preserve the ornaments.
13. Tie a string through the hole of each ornament.

## Scented Gift Ornaments

When you give these ornaments as gifts, attach a note to each one saying that it is to be hung in a closet to give off a wonderful scent. They are also nice to hang from the rearview mirror to give a car a pleasing aroma.

1 cup cinnamon
1 tablespoon ground cloves
1 tablespoon nutmeg
¾ cup applesauce
2 tablespoons white glue (Elmer's glue is gluten- and dairy-free)
Cookie cutters (optional)
1 toothpick
Ribbon

1. In a medium bowl, stir together the cinnamon, cloves, and nutmeg.
2. Stir in the applesauce and glue.
3. With your hands, knead the dough for 3 minutes or until the dough is smooth and all the ingredients are well blended.
4. Working with small batches of dough, roll out each batch to ¼-inch thickness.
5. Use cookie cutters to cut the dough into desired shapes.
6. Use a toothpick to make a small hole near the top of each ornament.
7. Place the ornaments on a wire rack. Allow them to dry for several days at room temperature. Turn the ornaments over each day so they dry evenly.
8. Thread a piece of ribbon through each hole for hanging.

## Face Paint

Painting faces is fun, whether you are the clown for a backyard circus, dressing up for Halloween, or just playing with friends.

2 teaspoons solid vegetable shortening

5 teaspoons cornstarch

1 teaspoon gluten-free flour mixture (See the Gluten-Free Flour Mixtures on page 16)

Glycerin (available at pharmacies)

Food coloring (optional)

1. Put the shortening, cornstarch, and flour mixture in a small bowl. Stir with a small spoon to form a smooth paste. Add 3 or 4 drops of glycerin for a creamy texture.
2. The mixture you now have will be a wonderful white that you may apply. But if you wish to color your paint, divide the mixture into several different small bowls and stir two drops of food coloring into each bowl.

## Eggseptional Garden

The eggs in this garden can have either straight hair (using grass) or curly hair (using parsley).

1 egg
Felt-tipped markers
1 empty egg carton
Potting soil
Grass seed (or parsley seed)
Water mister

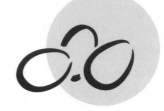

1. Carefully crack the egg in half over a bowl, letting the egg white and yolk drop into the bowl. (Cover the bowl with plastic wrap and refrigerate the insides of the egg to be used in a different recipe.) Rinse out both halves of the shell, then dry them very carefully so you don't break them.

2. Hold each half of the eggshell with the rounded end at the bottom and paint a funny face on it using markers. (Don't press too hard or the shell will break.)

3. Place the halves in the egg carton or in an egg holder.

4. Gently fill each half shell with potting soil. Sprinkle grass seeds or parsley seeds on top of the soil. Water the seeds with a water mister, or very lightly sprinkle with water.

5. Place near a sunny window, and watch your garden grow.

6. When the faces you drew on your eggs look like they have a full head of hair, plant the egg heads in your garden outside, shell and all.

# Marbleized Easter Eggs

Aluminum foil

1 roll paper towels

1 box assorted food coloring

6 hard-boiled eggs

1. Tear off a sheet of aluminum foil a bit bigger than 1 sheet of paper toweling. Place the foil on a protected work surface (for example, on top of a cutting board).
2. Place one paper towel on top of the foil.
3. Put 8 to 10 drops of food coloring (one or more colors) in the center of the paper towel. Allow a few minutes for the color to spread about 6 inches in diameter.
4. Place a damp (but not too wet) egg on its side in the center of the paper towel. Starting at the bottom of the egg, very gently press the foil around the egg, working your fingers toward the top, until the egg is completely wrapped.
5. Carefully peel back the foil and paper towel together. Remove the egg and let it dry. The effects will vary according to the colors used and the folds in the foil.

# Sugar Igloo

100 sugar cubes

5-inch cardboard circle

3 egg whites

2½ cups powdered sugar

1. Lay a base row of sugar cubes around the edge of the cardboard, leaving a space for the igloo entrance.
2. Make glue by mixing the egg whites with enough powdered sugar in a small bowl to form a paste. Add a few drops of water if the glue gets too thick to work with.

③ Spread a little bit of paste on the bottom of a sugar cube, and set the cube on top of the first row of sugar cubes. Continue with more sugar cubes, staggering the cubes so they do not line up exactly with the ones on the layer below. Complete a second row, keeping the entrance of the igloo open.

④ Continue building rows with the paste and sugar cubes. With each row, set the cubes a little closer to the center of the circle so that you form the shape of an igloo!

⑤ After five layers, let the cubes dry for several hours before adding more layers. There should be a total of ten layers.

⑥ Make the doorway arch separately by laying the sugar cubes into the shape of an arch and pasting them together. When the arch is dry, paste it in place, forming the doorway to the igloo.

⑦ Allow the completed igloo to dry overnight.

## Vinegar Painting

Red tissue paper
¼ cup white vinegar
1 thin paintbrush
White construction paper

① Cut small heart shapes from the tissue paper.

② Pour the vinegar into a small bowl.

③ Brush vinegar over an area of the construction paper. Lay a tissue paper heart over the brushed area. Repeat this process with the remaining hearts.

④ As the vinegar dries, the tissue paper will fall off, leaving red heart prints on the construction paper.

**Note:** Different colors of paper can be used for different seasons: for fall, cut brown tissue paper into the shape of leaves. For spring, cut orange and green tissue paper into the shapes of flowers and leaves.

## Building Blocks

You can create colorful blocks by mixing the marshmallows with boxes of various gluten-free gelatins in large, reclosable plastic bags.

> Toothpicks with rounded edges
> Marshmallows, large or small (Sweet & Sara brand marshmallows are gluten- and dairy-free)

1. Insert toothpicks into the marshmallows to create your own building blocks.
2. Connect the marshmallows to construct different types of buildings, such as castles, igloos, or forts. Use your imagination!

## Bean Sprouts

Bean sprouts are edible. Try adding them to salads.

> 1 paper towel
> 1 reclosable, sandwich-size plastic bag
> Water
> 4 dried beans

1. Place the paper towel inside the plastic bag.
2. Add just enough water to dampen the paper towel.
3. Add the beans to the bag. Seal the bag and store it in a dark place for four days, adding a few drops of water to the bag if the paper towel gets dry.
4. Once the sprouts appear, open the bag and place it on a windowsill where it can get sunlight.
5. When the sprouts are ½ inch long, transfer them to a shallow dish. Sprinkle them lightly with water each day. In about a week, the sprouts should be ready for harvesting.

## Bird Feeder

Hang this bird feeder close to the house during the winter so you can watch the birds feed.

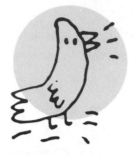

Cookie cutter (optional)
1 slice gluten-free bread (Ener-G
    Foods Tapioca Bread is gluten-
    and dairy-free)
1 toothpick
String
2 tablespoons peanut butter
3 tablespoons birdseed

1. Using a cookie cutter, cut out a shape from the center of the bread.
2. Let the bread shape dry for two days in the open air.
3. With a toothpick, poke a hole near the top of the bread shape.
4. Thread a piece of string through the hole.
5. Spread both sides of the bread with peanut butter.
6. Sprinkle both sides with birdseed.
7. Hang the bird feeder from a tree or a fence, tying the strings around a branch or fence post.

## Milk Painting

You can decorate bread for holidays and special occasions using Easter egg, pumpkin, or heart designs. What makes it fun is that it's edible!

2 tablespoons milk (use casein-free soy or rice milk for dairy-free
    diets)
2 (3-ounce) paper cups
1 drop each of 2 different food colorings
1 new, thin paintbrush
1 slice gluten-free bread (Kinnikinnick White Bread is gluten- and
    dairy-free)

1. Pour 1 tablespoon of milk into each of the paper cups.
2. Put 1 drop of food coloring into one cup and 1 drop of the other food coloring into the other cup.
3. Using a new, thin paintbrush, paint the bread with a design or your name. (Don't use so much milk-paint that your bread becomes soggy.)
4. Toast your bread, and see the finished creation!

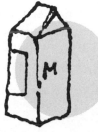

## Ĕggshell Art

Spring is a great time to make this project using colorful eggshells from Easter.

Eggshells
Felt-tipped markers or crayons
1 piece of paper
Glue (Elmer's glue is gluten- and dairy-free)
Paint (Crayola paints are gluten-free)

1. Whenever you or someone else uses an egg for cooking, save the shell. Rinse it well, and then lay it on paper towels till it is completely dry. Store the shells in a reclosable plastic bag.
2. Break the dried eggshells into tiny bits.
3. With markers or crayons, draw simple pictures on a piece of paper (for example, a kite, flower, fish, teddy bear, or plane).
4. Spread glue inside the outlined picture.
5. Sprinkle the bits of broken eggshells onto the glue. Allow this to dry for 2 hours. You can then paint the eggshells after the glue has dried.

## Gumdrop Christmas Tree

Vary the size of the trees you create by using large gluten-free gumdrops.

　　1 box toothpicks
　　1 bag small gluten-free gumdrops
　　1 (10-inch) Styrofoam cone

1　Push a toothpick into the bottom of a gumdrop. Push the other end into the side of the cone, starting near the bottom. (If you start at the top, the cone will get top-heavy and fall over.)

2　Continue attaching gumdrops, working your way up the cone, until the cone is covered in gumdrops.

## Candy Wreath

Make a candy wreath for every season!

　　1 sturdy wire coat hanger
　　Masking tape
　　Curling ribbon
　　2 pounds assorted wrapped gluten-free hard candies

1　Unbend the coat hanger and shape it into an 8-inch circle. Twist the wire around the top, leaving the hook intact.

2　Wrap the entire circle with masking tape. (This keeps the curling ribbon from slipping.)

3　With a 2-inch piece of curling ribbon, tie one end of a candy tightly to the wreath. Continue doing this, tying candies in different directions so they form a semicircle around the wire, until the circle is tightly covered with candies.

4　Wrap ribbon around the top of the hanger. Tie a bow at the bottom of the hook.

**Note:** You can use root beer and butterscotch candies with yellow and black ribbon for Halloween. Pink and yellow ribbons can be paired with individually wrapped, gluten-free, pastel jelly candies for spring.

## Marshmallow Snowman

You can create a family of snowmen by using miniature marshmallows to make the children.

5 toothpicks
3 large marshmallows (Sweet & Sara brand marshmallows are
    gluten- and dairy-free)
Orange felt-tipped marker
Gluten-free decorating gel
1 semisweet chocolate piece

1. Push a toothpick halfway into the center of a marshmallow. Place a second marshmallow on top of the first, pushing the other half of the toothpick through it to hold it in place. Push a second toothpick halfway through the top of the second marshmallow. Place the third marshmallow on top of the second, pushing the other half of the toothpick through to hold it in place.

2. Use broken pieces of toothpicks for the arms. For the snowman's nose, you can use a broken toothpick, using a marker to color it orange. Insert it into the top marshmallow for the nose. Use decorating gel to make the eyes, mouth, and buttons.

3. Put a little glob of decorating gel on the top of the top marshmallow, then place the chocolate piece on the gel for a hat. (Once the gel sets, it will act as glue and hold the "hat" on.)

## Homemade Barrettes

This craft project calls for the use of a glue gun, so it requires adult supervision.

> Small holiday candy (for example, candy corn for fall, candy hearts
>     for Valentine's Day, jelly beans for Easter)
> 1 metal barrette (available at craft stores)
> Sponge-type "paintbrush"
> Clear polyurethane
> String

1. Using a glue gun, hot-glue candies onto the barrette.
2. With the sponge brush, cover the candies completely with polyurethane. Thread a piece of string through the barrette and hang it from the bottom of a hanger. Hang the hanger in a well-ventilated open space. Let the barrette dry 24 hours.
3. Apply a second coat of polyurethane. Let it dry 24 hours.

**Note:** If the completed project is coated with polyurethane, the barrettes should last for years.

## Potpourri

For variety, you can add miniature pinecones, bay leaves, dried leaves, and petals from other flowers to your potpourri.

> 3 cups fresh rose petals
> 1 tablespoon ground cloves
> 1 tablespoon nutmeg
> 1 tablespoon cinnamon
> 2 tablespoons brown sugar

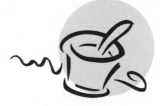

1. Spread rose petals in a single layer on paper towels. Let them dry for 1 week.
2. In a bowl, gently mix the dried petals with the cloves, nutmeg, cinnamon, and brown sugar.
3. To scent a room, place the mixture in a bowl. To scent a drawer, place in a small fabric bag, or lay it on several layers of tulle netting, then bring the sides together and tie with a ribbon.

## Pictures from the Kitchen

Kitchen supplies are perfect to use when making scenic collages or for other fun pictures. Draw your picture first with crayons, and then enhance the picture by gluing kitchen supplies on top. Use any of the following items for your project, or let your imagination run wild.

> A cinnamon stick for a tree trunk and bay leaves for the leaves of
> the tree
> Toothpicks for fences
> Sesame seeds for a gravel driveway
> Small elbow macaroni (gluten-free, of course) for a tile roof
> Red candy hearts for flowers
> Fresh coffee grounds or cocoa for dirt
> Foil for a frozen pond or ice-skating rink
> Blue plastic wrap for pool water
> Powdered sugar or cotton balls for clouds
> Eggshells for house siding
> Cut-up napkins for curtains

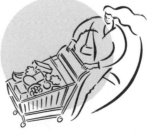

# index

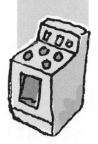